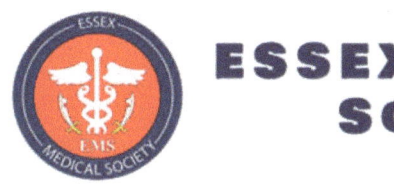

ESSEX MEDICAL SOCIETY

PHYSICAL DIAGNOSIS
SIGNS AND HISTORY TAKING

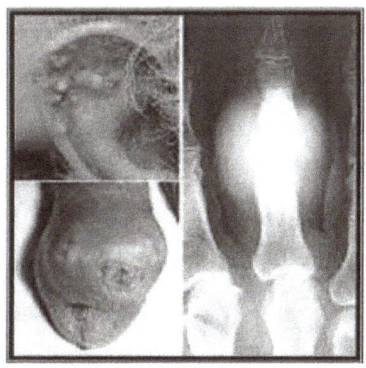

COMPILED BY

Professor Tham Nimal-Raj

Mr Peter Smith

Professor S Sampathkumar

A compilation of facts from various sources for educational purposes.

Published by New Generation Publishing in 2021

Copyright © T Nimal-Raj 2021

The authors assert the moral right under the Copyright, Designs and Patents Act 1988 to be identified as the authors of this work.

All Rights reserved. No part of this publication may be reproduced, stored in a retrieval system or transmitted, in any form or by any means without the prior consent of the authors, nor be otherwise circulated in any form of binding or cover other than that which it is published and without a similar condition being imposed on the subsequent purchaser.

www.newgeneration-publishing.com

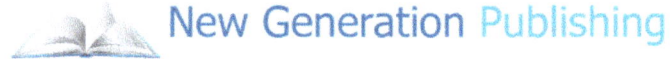

PREFACE

Professor NIMAL-RAJ

Has been a teacher for postgraduate and undergraduate medical students in Anatomy & Primary Care.

An avid teacher and mentor, he mentors senior doctors and advises many institutions and organizations.

This is his third book and there are four books in the making for the year 2020/2021.

All revenue from the books will be given to charity.

Professor S. SAMPATHKUMAR

Studied Medicine and Anaesthesia in India and moved to UK in 1994. Obtained CCST in anaesthesia and became a Consultant Anaesthetist at Basildon & Thurrock University Hospitals NHS Trust in 2001. Currently I am working as a senior consultant in Anaesthesia.

I am an accomplished and high-achieving medical professional, with compelling success, managing patients as a Senior Consultant Anaesthetist. Exceptional knowledge and experience in Trauma and Elective Major Orthopaedics, Vascular anaesthesia, urology, major gastro intestinal surgery, spine surgery, Acute pain management and peri operative medicine. Developed an interest in applied physics in Medicine and basic sciences in Anaesthesia. Have an interest in teaching students. Worked in different positions like College Tutor, Anaesthetic Service Unit Lead, Lead for Trauma and enhanced recovery. Excellent communication, presentation and diplomacy skills, with a proven ability to build long lasting trust, and mutual respect at all levels.

I have contributed to many people to publish books with materials, sharing clinical information and other supports. I thank all those who provided me with pictures and other materials for this book. A special note to mention Professor Tham Nimal-Raj, who is an inspiration to me and always there for support.

Medical students – this is a short compilation of facts made easy to refer and refresh your reading mind. This is to enhance knowledge and rapid reflection of what has been taught, and is useful to junior and senior doctors.

It is an art and science to capture the syndromes and myriad of disease patterns.

This is a collection from various medical materials.

We hope that peers will enjoy this book.

Regards,
Authors

MAIN AUTHOR

Professor Tham Nimal-Raj

Provost & Professor at New Vision University TBLISI, Republic of Georgia.
Senior Primary Care Physician in NHS UK.
East Tilbury Medical Centre, Tilbury Medical Centre, Corringham Health Centre, Thurrock CCG HUB,
Thurrock CCG Cancer Lead, & Unplanned Care Lead CCG NHS.
Private Primary Care Physician,
Queen Anne Street Medical Centre London

Linkedin: https://www.linkedin.com/in/nimal-raj
Email: Profraj7@gmail.com, Nimal.raj@nhs.net

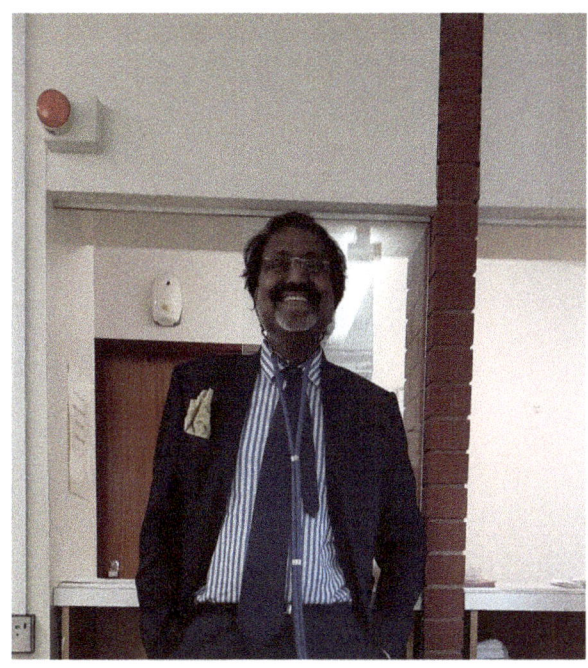

AUTHORS

Professor S. Sampathkumar

Illustrations,
Selections of medical images.

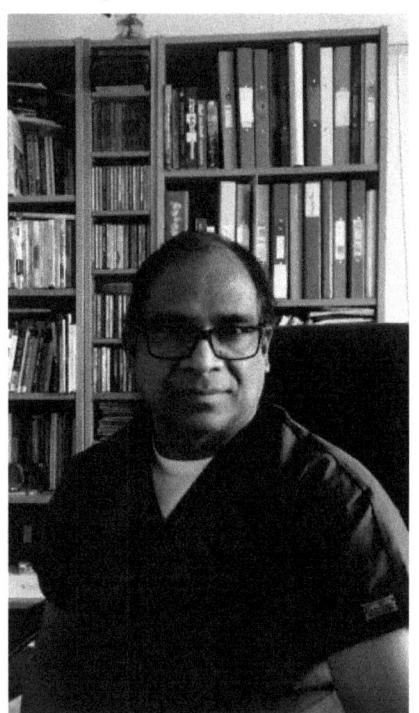

Also:

Peter Smith, BSc (Hons)
Senior Pharmaceutical industry specialist
Medical compiling and assisting,
Editorial Assistant.

MEDICAL STUDENTS CONTRIBUTION

Mr Deepaesh Sivalingham

Clinical Medical Student,
Riga Stradins University Medical School, Latvia, RSU.
Assisted with illustrations.

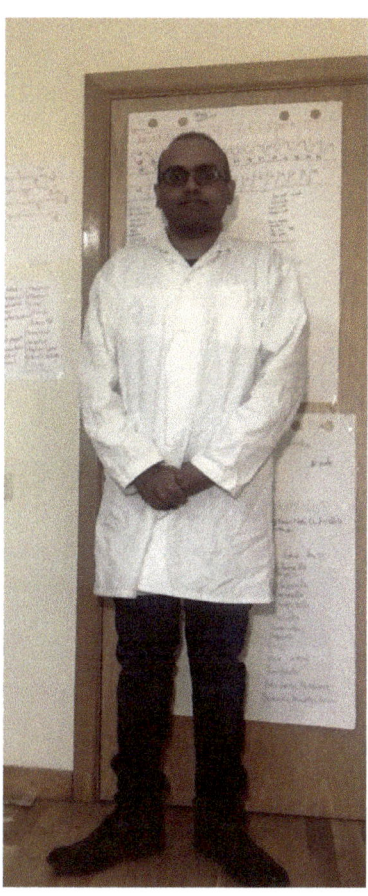

EDITORIAL SUPPORT

Mr Benaiah Osakwe

LLB (Hons),
Aston University

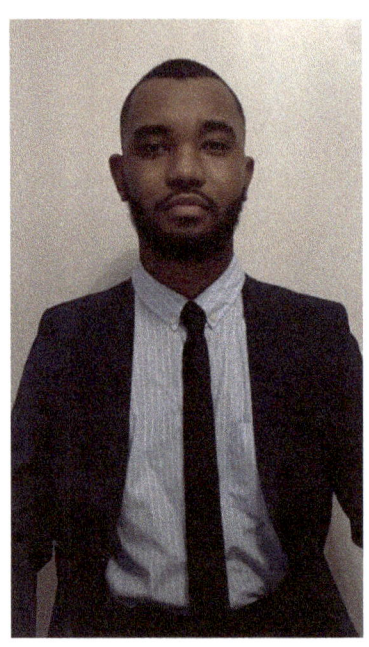

DEDICATION

We dedicate this to our teachers who have taught us with commitment and devotion to make us attain a standard of safety to deliver the best care for our patients.

We dedicate all revenue to Save The Children *charity.*

MICHELANGELO

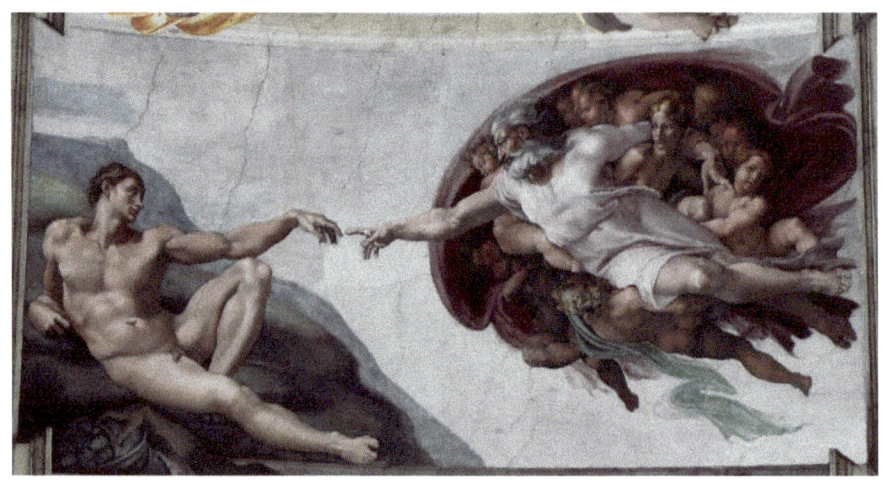

"THE ART & SCIENCE OF MEDICINE
CONSISTS OF AMUSING THE PATIENT
LIKE A MAGICIAN.

LEAVE THE NATURE TO CURE THE DISEASE.
SHOW WHILE IN PRACTICE
RESPECT & HUMILITY."

Prof. N. R. RAJ

CONTENTS

THE HISTORY AND PHYSICAL SYNOPSIS 17
    Chief Complaint 17
    History Of Present Illness 17
    Past Medical History 17
    Family History 17
    Personal/ Social History 17
    Review Of Systems 18
    Physical Exam 19
    Physical Diagnosis 22

1.0 HEAD AND NECK 22
    1.1 THE EYE 22
        Symptoms: 22
        Sudden Loss Of Vision 22
        Gradual Loss Of Vision 22
        Diplopia (Double Vision) 23
        Eye Pain 23
        Eyelids 24
        Sclera 24
        Cornea 25
        Pupils 26
        Extraocular Palsies 27
        Visual Field Deficits 27
        Funduscopic Inspection 28
    1.2 THE EAR 29
        Tinnitus: Ringing In Ear 29
        Vertigo 29
        Rinne Test 29
        Weber Test 29
        Meniere's Disease 29
        Benign Positional Vertigo 30
    1.3 NOSE AND THROAT 30
        Nose 30

	Throat	30
	Abnormal Taste	30
	Tongue	31
	Mouth Examination:	31
2.0	**RESPIRATORY SYSTEM**	33
	Pulmonary Symptoms	33
	Cough	33
	Sputum	33
	Hemoptysis	34
	Pleuritic Chest Pain	34
	Dyspnea	35
	Orthopnea	35
	Paroxysmal Nocturnal Dyspnea	35
	Wheezing	36
	Cyanosis	36
	Rhinorrhea	36
	Family / Social History	37
	Extrapulmonary Examination	37
	Breathing	38
	Inspection	38
	Palpation	39
	Pneumothorax	40
	Percussion	40
	Auscultation	41
	Lung Diseases	43
3.0	**CARDIAC**	44
	Cardiac Symptoms, History	44
	Chest Pain	44
	Angina (Ischemic Cardiac Pain)	44
	Non-Ischemic Cardiac Pain	45
	Pleuritic (Pulmonary) Chest Pain	45
	Gastrointestinal Chest Pain	46
	Chest Wall Pain	46
	Dyspnea	47

	Palpitations	48
	Fatigue	48
	Syncope	49
	Hemoptysis	50
	Edema	50
	Cyanosis	50
	General Physical Exam	51
	Blood Pressure	51
	Jugular Venous Pulses	52
	Arterial Pulses	54
	The Precordium	56
	PalPation / Percussion	56
	Stethoscope	57
	Heart Sounds	57
	Heart Murmurs: General Properties	59
	Systolic Murmurs	60
	Diastolic Murmurs	62
	Techniques For Enhancing Auscultation	64
4.0	**ABDOMEN**	**67**
	History Taking	67
	Abdominal Pain	67
	Anorexia	68
	Nausea And Vomiting	68
	Dysphagia	69
	Diarrhea	69
	Constipation	70
	Hematemesis	71
	Hematochezia And Melena	71
	Inspection	71
	Protuberant or Distended Abdomen	71
	Grey Turner's Sign	72
	Jaundice	72
	Abdominal Hernias	73
	Percussion	74

	Auscultation	74
	Palpation	75
	Liver	75
	Spleen	75
	Gallbladder	75
	Kidneys	75
	Aorta	76
	Masses And Bowel Loops	76
	Femoral Pulses And Distal Aorta	76
	Rectal Exam	76
	Acute Abdominal Pain	76
	Direct And Indirect Tenderness	77
	Abdominal Pain Syndromes	77
	Acute Abdominal Pain	77
	Chronic Abdominal Pain	77
	Anterior Abdominal Wall Pain	78
5.0	**MALE GENITALIA**	79
	Symptoms	79
	Physical Exam	80
	Penis	80
	Scrotum	81
	Prostate	81
	Inguinal Canals And Groin	81
	Rectal Exam	81
6.0	**FEMALE GENITALIA**	82
	Symptoms	82
	Past History	82
	Abnormalities In Menstruation	82
	Other Things Relating To Menstruation	84
	Non-Menstrual Vaginal Bleeding	84
	Pelvic Pain	84
	Urinary Tract Infections	85
	Pregnancy And Infertility	85
	Abnormalities In Sexual Function	86

	Vaginal Discharge And Itching	87
	Pelvic Relaxation	88
	Hirsutism	88
	Physical Exam	88
7.0	**MUSCULOSKELETAL**	89
	Epidemiology	89
	Symptoms	89
	Reiter's Syndrome:	89
	Psoriatic Arthritis	90
	Gout	90
	Rheumatic Fever	90
	Gonorrhea, Disseminated	91
	Rheumatoid Arthritis	91
	Osteoarthritis	92
	Systemic Lupus Erythematosus	92
	Symptoms	93
	Pain	93
	Stiffness	93
	Weakness	93
	Inspection	93
	Palpation	93
	Deformity	94
	Erythema And Warmth	94
	Limitation Of Range Of Motion	94
	Tenderness	94
	Auscultation	95
	Muscle Strength	95
	Range Of Motion	95
	Head Exam	96
	Neck (Cervical Spine)	96
	Shoulder	96
	Elbow	96
	Wrist	97
	Spine	98

	Hip	98
	Knee	98
	Ankle and Feet	99
8.0	**NEUROLOGICAL**	100
	Neurologic Symptoms	100
	Headache	100
	Syncope and Loss of Consciousness	100
	Seizures	100
	Neurologic Exam:	103
	Assessment of Motor Function	103
	Motor Abnormalities:	103
	Sensory Evaluation	104
	Stereognosis	104
	Cerebellar Function	104
	Reflexes	105
	Deep Tendon Reflexes:	105
	Absence Of Superficial Reflexes	107
	Primitive Reflexes	107
	Cranial Nerve Evaluation:	107
	Physical Signs	111
TABLE OF PHYSICAL FINDINGS		115
ILLUSTRATIONS		123

THE HISTORY AND PHYSICAL SYNOPSIS

CHIEF COMPLAINT (CC):
The reason(s) for which the patient is visiting.

HISTORY OF PRESENT ILLNESS (HPI):
Chronological narrative of the circumstances leading up to the chief complaint(s). Discussion of associated complaints and the signs and symptoms of the chief complaint, but no diagnostic label.

PAST MEDICAL HISTORY (PMH):
1. Major illnesses
2. Injuries
3. Operations
4. Immunization history
5. Allergies to medication, food, contact, asthma
6. Dates of last chest X-ray and PAP smear; results?
7. Use of medications? Non-prescription, prescription, birth-control pills, caffeine, recreational, smoking

FAMILY HISTORY (FH): Father, mother: Age or age at death, cause of death, illnesses they have had; cancer, heart-disease, diabetes, stroke, alcoholism; history of illness of all primary relatives.

PERSONAL/ SOCIAL HISTORY (SH): Place of birth, residence, occupation, marital status, number/ age / sex of all children, brief description of lifestyle and eating and sleeping habits, travel, religion.

1. **Tobacco (package-years), alcohol, recreational drugs consumption.**
2. **Sexual History:** Sexual trauma (rape, incest), sexually active, male homosexuality, multiple partners, risk-factors for STD's and AIDS, contraception, satisfaction with sex life.

REVIEW OF SYSTEMS (ROS):
Interview patient about somatic systems.

1. **General:** *Height, weight, appetite, fatigue, weakness, chills, night sweats, anorexia, syncope, insomnia*
2. **Skin:** *Colour change, itching, rashes, dryness, moles, infections, tumours*
3. **Head:** *Headaches, trauma*
4. **Eyes:** *Itching, redness, vision, glasses, blindness or blind spots, glaucoma, burning, dryness.*
5. **Ears:** *Hearing, vertigo, earaches, discharge, tinnitus.*
6. **Nose/ Sinuses:** *Bleeding, dryness, discharge, obstruction, pain, sinusitis.*
7. **Mouth:** *Dental caries, bleeding gum, sore tongue, post-nasal drip.*
8. **Throat:** *Hoarseness, painful swallowing, tonsillitis.*
9. **Neck:** *Stiffness, pain, decreased motion, lumps, swollen glands, goitre.*

1. **Breasts:** *Pain, tenderness, lumps, nipple discharge.*
2. **Respiratory:** *Exertional dyspnea, cough, sputum, hemoptysis, wheezing, TB Test, recurrent respiratory infections.*
3. **Cardiac:** *Angina, orthopnea, paroxysmal nocturnal dyspnea, murmur, palpitations, syncope.*
4. **Vascular:** *Varicosities, Raynaud's (cold-exposed pallor, cyanosis, redness).*
5. **Gastrointestinal:** *Nausea, vomiting, dysphagia, heartburn, hematemesis, haemorrhoids, blood in stool, constipation, food intolerances.*
6. **Urinary Tract:** *Hematuria, dysuria, burning, incontinence, history of infections, polyuria, nocturia.*
7. **Female Reproductive:** *Age at menarche, menorrhagia, postcoital bleeding, vaginal discharge, obstetrical history (miscarriages, gravida, para), libido, contraceptive use, menstrual regularity, dysmenorrhea.*
8. **Male Reproductive:** *Penile discharge, pain, history of venereal disease, libido, infertility, impotence, testicular pain or masses.*
9. **Hematologic:** *anaemia, easy bruising, easy bleeding,*

bleeding gums, lymphadenopathy.
10. **Musculoskeletal:** *Muscle pain, weakness, joints, abnormal curvature (kyphosis, lordosis).*
11. **Endocrine:** *Heat/ Cold intolerance, breath change, voice change, Diabetes (polydipsia, polyuria, polyphagia).*
12. **Central Nervous System:** *Headache, syncope, seizures, vertigo, blindness, diplopia (double-vision), tremor, ataxia, memory, numbness, paresthesia.*
13. **Psychiatric:** *Nervousness, depression, hyperventilation, insomnia, phobias, emotional instability, delusions.*

PHYSICAL EXAM (PE)
1. **Vital Signs**
    1. Temperature
    2. Respiratory Rate
    3. Pulse
    4. Blood Pressure
    5. Height
    6. Weight
2. **General Appearance:** *Nutrition, body habitus, apparent age, colour, general behaviour.*
3. **Skin:** *Dry, coarse, smooth, rashes and scars (indicate position), temperature, baldness, hair, abnormal pigmentations, needle tracks, bruises, hirsutism.*
4. **Lymph Nodes:** *Enlargement, tenderness; anterior+ posterior cervical, axillary, inguinal, femoral. Record size in cm if enlarged.*
5. **Head:** *Size, shape, symmetry, contour, tenderness, bruits; anterior fontanelle (ped).*
6. **Eyes:** *Conjunctiva, sclerae, pupil size and reaction, ptosis, protrusion, gross visual acuity, extraocular movements, visual fields, pupillary light and accommodation reflexes; Funduscopic: optic disc, fovea, pupil/edema.*
7. **Ears:** *Tympanic membrane, discharge, cerumen, hearing, Weber test, Rinne test.*
8. **Nose:** *Septum, mucosa, airway obstruction, discharge, polyps*
9. **Mouth and Throat:** *Odour of breath, colour of lips, tongue, and gums; caries, tonsils, uvula, larynx, epiglottis, anterior*

cervical and submaxillary nodes, carotid and jugular pulses.
10. **Breasts:** *Tenderness, lumps, gynecomastia, symmetry.*
11. **Back:** *Mobility, curvature, tenderness on palpation or percussion.*
12. **Thorax:** *General symmetry, movement with respiration.*
13. **Respiratory:**
    1. **Inspection:** *Laboured or shallow breathing, use of accessory respiratory muscles.*
    2. **Palpation:** *Palpate costochondral junction for areas of tenderness.*
    3. **Percussion:** *Dullness, hyperresonance, diaphragm excursion.*
    4. **Auscultation:** *Crackles, wheezes, rubs.*
14. **Heart:**
    1. **Inspection:** *Heaving, bulging, point of maximal impulse.*
    2. **Palpation:** *Costochondral junctions for tenderness.*
    3. **Percussion:** *Heart size*
    4. **Auscultation:** *Rate and rhythm of normal sounds at each of the valve locations, 53, 54, murmurs; draw diagrams indicating time and location of extra sounds.*
15. **Abdomen:**
    1. **Inspection:** *Obese, flat, distended, dilated veins, scars, hair distribution*
    2. **Palpation:** *Tenderness, rigidity, hernia, liver span, spleen palpable?*
    3. **Percussion:** *Organ size, dullness, tympany*
    4. **Auscultation:** *Bowel sounds, rubs, bruits*
16. **Extremities:** *Joint swelling, tenderness, edema, rashes; muscle weakness, hair distribution.*
17. **Vascular:** *Pulses (carotid, brachial, radial, femoral, popliteal, dorsalis pedis, posterior tibial). Use three-point scale to indicate magnitude of pulse.*
18. **Male Genitalia:** *Size/ tenderness of testis, urethral discharge, epididymis*
19. **Female Genitalia:**
    1. **External:** *Hair distribution, labia, clitoris, introitus, urethra*
    2. **Internal:** *Cervix, Cervical pain with motion, adnexa including ovaries, cul-de-sac, PAP smear, rectovaginal*

20. **Rectal:** *Prostate, faeces analysis, polyps or masses.*
21. **Neurological:**
    1. **Mental Status**
    2. **Cranial Nerves Tests**
    3. **Somatic Reflexes**
    4. **Motor:** *Muscular Strength, flaccidity I spasticity, tremor*
    5. **dystopia**
    6. **Cerebellar**: *Gait, finger-to-nose, finger-to-finger, Romberg Test*
    7. **Sensory**: *Dermatome distribution, two-point discrimination*

PHYSICAL DIAGNOSIS

1.0 HEAD and NECK

1.1 THE EYE

SYMPTOMS:

***SUDDEN LOSS of VISION:* Potential Causes**

- **AMAUROSIS FUGAX:** Temporary, monocular, ischemic blindness.
    - Painless
    - Caused by ipsilateral Carotid stenosis or embolization of the retinal artery.

- **RETINAL DETACHMENT:** Flashing lights, floating halos, and blurry vision before the blindness is indicative of retinal detachment.

- **UVEITIS:** Inflammation of uveal tract – iris, ciliary body, and choroid.
    - Always painful
    - Associated with multiple diseases: connective tissue diseases, histoplasmosis, sarcoidosis, tuberculosis.

***GRADUAL LOSS of VISION:* Potential Causes**

- **CATARACTS:** Opacities of the lens, occurring with age.

- **GLAUCOMA:** Increased intraocular pressure.
    - *It is the most common reason for loss of vision over age 50.*

- **MACULAR DEGENERATION:** Secondary to Diabetes and expected to cause visual blindness.
    - *Diabetic Retinopathy.*

- **OPTIC NERVE COMPRESSION:** Caused by an intracranial neoplasm, or pituitary adenoma.

- **OPTIC NEUROPATHY (Optic Neuritis):** Multiple Sclerosis, and drugs such as Ethambutol and Methanol can cause optic neuritis and gradual blindness.

- **PRESBYOPIA:** Gradual loss of ability of Accommodation for near-vision, occurring with age.

- **CORTICAL BLINDNESS:** Infarct of the Occipital Lobe can lead to cortical blindness. Patient will have binocular blindness but will retain the pupillary light reflex which is unaffected.

DIPLOPIA (Double vision): **Potential causes**

- **MONOCULAR DIPLOPIA:** Should suggest corneal or lens problem.

- **BINOCULAR DIPLOPIA:** Indicative of cranial nerve palsy or ocular muscle problems, or a brainstem problem.

- **MYASTHENIA GRAVIS (MG):** Diplopia without pain is often the presenting complaint in MG.

EYE PAIN:

- The cornea is innervated by the **Ophthalmic Nerve, CN vi.**

- Potential causes of eye pain:

    o CNS problems affecting CN V^1: Meningitis, cavernous sinus thrombosis, aneurysms, migraine

    o Adjacent structures: sinus problems

    o Eye problems/ inflammations: Conjunctivitis, stye, chalazion

- **PHOTOPHOBIA:** Eye pain upon exposure to light, indicative of:

- **SCOTOMATA:** Specific islands or spots of impaired vision; an impaired visual field.

EYELIDS:

- **PTOSIS:** Droopy eyelids; failure of lids to open fully.
    - Caused by failure of levator palpebrae, innervated by CN III, or failure of Tarsal Muscle, innervated by sympathetics.
    - Some causes: Homer's Syndrome, Myasthenia Gravis, Encephalitis

- **LID LAG:** Evidence of white sclera between the iris and upper lid margin. This is normally not found.
    - It is a sign of Grave's Disease

- **STYE:** Small abscess caused by infection of sebaceous glands of Zeis.

- **CHALAZION:** Acute inflammation of the meibomian gland.

SCLERA:

- **SCLERITIS:** Inflammation of the sclera, visible as brown / red infiltrates in sclera on gross examination. Found in autoimmune and collagen vascular diseases, such as SLE, RA.

- **BLUE SCLERA:** Pathognomonic of Osteogenesis Imperfecta.
    - Results from very thin sclera in which the choroid shows through.

- **BROWN SCLERA:** Found in disorder Alkaptonuria (metabolic disorder).

- **YELLOW SCLERA:** Found in *Jaundice*. It should raise the question of liver disease or hemolytic anaemia.

- **EXOPHTHALMOS:** Eyes jutting out past eyelids. A sign of Grave's disease, acromegaly, and cavernous sinus thrombosis.

CORNEA:

- **KERATOCONJUNCTIVITIS (KERATITIS) SICCA:** Found in **Sjogren's Syndrome**, resulting from autoantibodies against salivary glands resulting in no salivary secretion.

  o Classic triad of symptoms with Sjogren's Syndrome:

  - Keratitis Sicca (dry eyes)
  - Xerostomia (dry mouth)
  - Rheumatoid Arthritis

- **INTERSTITIAL KERATITIS:** A sign of congenital syphilis.

  o **Hutchinson's Triad:** Triad of interstitial keratitis, deafness, and notched teeth is classical evidence for congenital syphilis.

- **ARCUS SENILIS:** Gray band of opacity around the cornea.

- **KAYSER-FLEISCHER RINGS:** Copper in Descemet's Membrane.

  o Circular bands of brownish pigment on lateral and medial margins of cornea.

  o Found in **Wilson's Disease**.

- **PINGUECULAE:** Small, yellowish elevations of the conjunctivae, which appear brown in Gaucher's disease. It is caused by hyaline degeneration of conjunctival tissue.

- **ANISOCORIA: Unequal pupils,** caused by miosis or mydriasis of one pupil.

PUPILS:

- **MARCUS GUNN PUPIL:** A pupil that dilates (rather than constricts) as light swings toward it.
    - It indicates either severe macular disease or optic nerve disease in the affected eye.

- **PUPILLARY REFLEXES:**
    - Absent Direct Reflex: Indicates a problem with the afferent branch (Trigeminal V1) of the reflex.
    - Absent Consensual Reflex: Indicates a problem with the efferent branch (CN III, Edinger-Westphal Nucleus) of the affected eye.

- **CONVERGENCE:** Ability of eyes to focus inward and accommodate for near vision.
    - Impaired convergence is seen with Grave's Disease.

- **ARGYLL ROBERTSON PUPIL:** Indicates a form of CNS Syphilis, **Tabes Dorsalis.**
    - Weak or absent direct pupillary reflex.
    - Normal response to accommodation.
    - Failure of pupillary dilation with painful stimulation or after atropine administration.

- **ADIE'S PUPIL:** Similar to Argyll Robertson Pupil.
    - Weak or absent direct pupillary reflex.
    - Impaired or absent accommodation.
    - Eye appears larger than the other eye on inspection.

- **MYDRIASIS:** Abnormal dilation of pupil, can occur in Diabetes.

- **MIOSIS:** Abnormal constriction of pupil, seen in Homer's syndrome.

    o **HORNER'S SYNDROME**: Lost sympathetics from the Superior Cervical Plexus. Ptosis, Miosis, Anhydrosis.

- **NYSTAGMUS:** Nystagmus is normal when looking in the periphery for extended times. All other nystagmus is abnormal.

- CAUSES: Labyrinthitis, MS, Wernicke-Korsakoff, Meniere's Disease

EXTRAOCULAR PALSIES:

- **INTERNAL STRABISMUS:** Eye points in, due to denervation of the Abducens, CN VI.

- **EXTERNAL STRABISMUS**: Eye points out and down, due to denervation of the Oculomotor, CN III.

    o Eye points out because of influence of Abducens (CN VI)

    o Eye points down because of influence of Trochlear (CN IV) --------> Superior Oblique muscle.

VISUAL FIELD DEFICITS:

- **BITEMPORAL HEMIANOPSIA:** Loss of peripheral vision; tunnel vision, occurs with Pituitary Tumour.

- **HOMONYMOUS HEMIANOPSIA:** Loss of same visual field in both eyes. Occurs due to lesion in Optic Tract.

- **QUADRANT HEMIANOPSIA:** Lesion in the optic radiations.

FUNDUSCOPIC INSPECTION:

- **RED REFLEX:** Its absence indicates a cataract.

- **VESSELS**

    o   The veins are normally slightly bigger than the arteries.

    o   **ARTERIO-VENOUS (AV) NICKING:** Hypertension narrows the arteries and creates indentations in the veins, where arteries cross the veins.

- **MACULA:** Dimmer, darker area in fundoscope, containing the fovea.

- **OPTIC DISC:** Out of which vessels travel. The brightest area of fundoscope.

- **RETINOPATHOLOGIES:**

    o   **DIABETIC RETINOPATHY:** Shows hard exudates on the retina, which are lipid laden. They are dense, well-defined creamy white spots.

    - Cotton Wool Exudates are poorer defined and can occur with hypertension.

    o   **PAPILLEDEMA:** Swelling of retinal vessels, from impaired venous return in the eye ------> venous distension.

    - Papilledema is caused by increased intracranial pressure.
    - Causes: Brain tumours, malignant hypertension, hydrocephalus.
    - As opposed to Pappilitis, there is no loss of vision.

    o   **HYPERTENSION:** Changes in retina are graded 1 through 4. An abnormally high V/A ratio can be found, indicating venous distension.

    - Stage I: Arteriolar narrowing but no AV-nicking.

- Stage II: Focal spasm, AV-nicking.
- Stage III: Haemorrhages and exudates
- Stage IV: Papilledema, Optic disc edema (due to ischemia) and haemorrhage, which can lead to retinal detachment.

1.2 THE EAR

TINNITUS: Ringing in ear.

VERTIGO:

- Objective Vertigo: The earth is moving around you.
- Subjective Vertigo: You are moving in space.

RINNE TEST: Test for conductive hearing loss by comparing air conduction to bone conduction.

- First hold tuning fork right near auricle, then place it over the Mastoid Process.
- NORMAL: It should sound louder near the auricle, because air conduction should be better than straight bone conduction.
- ABNORMAL: If it sounds louder over the mastoid process instead, that indicates a conductive hearing loss in the middle ear.

WEBER TEST: Place tuning fork over head. It should be heard equally in both ears.

- ONE EAR IS LOUDER: If one ear is louder, than there is either conductive hearing loss in that ear or sensorineural hearing loss in the other ear.

MENIERE'S DISEASE: Triad of tinnitus, vertigo, and sensorineural hearing loss. May see nausea, vomiting, nystagmus.

BENIGN POSITIONAL VERTIGO: Transient attacks of vertigo, induced by movements of the head and trunk. Symptoms can be induced by having the patient merely think about the movements.

1.3   NOSE AND THROAT

NOSE:

- **EPISTAXIS (Bloody nose):**

    o   Transient Epistaxis: May occur with forceful nose-blowing, sneezing, nose-picking, facial trauma.

- **Recurrent Epistaxis:** Differential diagnosis

    o   hypertension, coagulopathies, renal failure, cirrhosis, hereditary haemorrhagic telangiectasia.

- **RHINOPHYMA:** Severe acne rosacea found in association with skin hypertrophy and congestion of subcutaneous tissue, around the nose.

THROAT:

- **SORE THROAT:** Infection mononucleosis, strep-throat (streptococcal pharyngitis).

- **HOARSENESS:** Laryngitis, Laryngeal cancer, hypothyroidism, smoking ------> broncho-genic carcinoma.

ABNORMAL TASTE:

- **HYPOGUESIA:** Impaired ability to taste. Seen in URI's, glossitis, stomatitis.

- **DYSGUESIA:** Unpleasant taste. Differential diagnosis:

    o   Medications: metronidazole

    o   Vitamin and mineral deficiencies: zinc depletion

- Chronic hypercalcemia, hyperparathyroidism.
- Viral hepatitis

TONGUE:

- **MACROGLOSSIA:**

  - Large tongue can occur with amyloidosis and acromegaly.

- **GLOSSITIS:** Inflammation on sides, base, and underside of tongue.

  - Vitamin and mineral deficiencies
  - Medications: metronidazole, phenytoin
  - Infections: candidiasis
  - Pernicious Anaemia
  - Cytotoxic drugs, radiotherapy.

MOUTH EXAMINATION:

- **ORAL ULCERS:** Recurrent oral ulcers differential diagnosis:

  - **Recurrent aphthous ulcers** (canker sores): Common, frequently associated with Inflammatory Bowel Disease.
  - Infections: **HSV-1,** Herpes Zoster, tuberculosis, histoplasmosis, syphilis.
  - Trauma
  - Cytotoxic drugs
  - Rare: Erythema Multiforme, Wegener's Granulomatosis, Stevens-Johnson Syndrome, Reiter's Syndrome

- **SYNDROMES:**

  o **PEUTZ-JEGHER'S SYNDROME:** Melanin spots on lips are found.

  o **OLIVER-WEBER-RENDU SYNDROME:** **Telangiectasia,** vascular lesion formed by dilation of small group of blood vessels

- **KOPLIK'S SPOTS:** White spots on the buccal mucosa, indicative of the measles.

- **STRAWBERRY TONGUE:** Erythema of tongue, occurs with scarlet fever.

2.0 RESPIRATORY SYSTEM

PULMONARY SYMPTOMS:

COUGH:

- **Possible Causes of Cough**:
  - Pulmonary/ Mechanical causes: Asthma, Irritants, aspiration.
  - Infectious: Tuberculosis, Histoplasmosis, Pneumonia.
  - Temperature: Inhaling cold air.
  - Pulmonary Embolism, pulmonary edema.
  - Non-Pulmonary: external ear canal irritation.

- **Details:**
  - **Smoker's Cough** usually occurs in the morning and is productive.
  - **Asthmatic Cough** usually is non-productive.

SPUTUM: It is always abnormal.

- **PRODUCTIVE COUGHS** are seen in:
  - Chronic Bronchitis, Smoker's cough.
  - **Bronchiectasis:** chronically dilated bronchioles.
  - Large volume of sputum, which separates into two or three layers upon standing.
- Tumours: Bronchoalveolar Carcinoma
- Infections: Pneumonia, Tuberculosis, Lung Abscess
  - Will usually see **yellow or green** sputum.
- Pulmonary Edema

HEMOPTYSIS:

CAUSES:

- Most common: Bronchitis, Bronchogenic Carcinoma, Pneumococcal Pneumonia
- More rare infections:
    - **Tuberculosis**: Age over 60, crackles, few other symptoms
    - Coccidiomycosis, Histoplasmosis
- Other tumours: Weight loss, cigarettes, anorexia
- Rare Immune Disorders: Goodpasture's Syndrome, Wegener's Granulomastosis
- **Pulmonary Embolism:**
    - High V/Q Ratio. Lots of ventilation, poor perfusion. Excessive dead space.
    - Friction rub, accentuated P2.
    - Pleuritic chest pain.
- **MASSIVE HEMOPTYSIS** = 600 ml in 24 hrs. Usually associated with bronchiectasis, and may be indicative of lung cancer or pulmonary aspergillosis.

PLEURITIC CHEST PAIN: Chest pain upon breathing.

- PULMONARY CAUSES: Bronchitis, pneumonia, pulmonary embolism, tuberculosis, lung carcinoma.
- NON-PULMONARY CAUSES:
    - Tietze's Syndrome (Costochondritis): Superficial chest pain with local tenderness.
    - Tracheitis presents with retrosternal chest pain, made worse by coughing.

DYSPNEA: Difficult, laboured breathing.

- Differential Diagnosis: A laundry list of possible causes:

    o Pulmonary Disease: COPD, cancer, asthma, chronic or acute bronchitis, emphysema, pneumonia, pulmonary emboli, pneumothorax
    o Cystic Fibrosis: Sweat test
    o Cardiac causes: CHF, Pulmonary edema, PND
    o Hematologic: Anemia, CO-Poisoning
    o Metabolic: Ketoacidosis
    o Salicylate poisoning

- Symptoms: Dyspnea may be masked by **tachypnea** (shallow, rapid breathing).

    o **Hyperpnea** is not tachypnea – it is hyperventilation (not laboured breathing) usually caused by metabolic acidosis and is unrelated to dyspnea. Distinguish the two with pulmonary function studies.

ORTHOPNEA: Dyspnea with onset occurring while lying down, and which is immediately corrected upon restoring upright position.
- Differential Diagnosis: **Congestive Heart Failure** or **COPD**

    o Also, bilateral paralysis of diaphragms.

***PAROXYSMAL NOCTURNAL DYSPNEA* (PND):**

- Dyspnea at night, created by lying down, but which does not immediately improve upon standing up. Patient feels acutely air-hungry and frequently wakes up at night. Night sweats common.

    o Differential Diagnosis: **Acute Pulmonary Edema** secondary to **congestive heart failure**.

WHEEZING: High-pitched musical breath sound usually heard on expiration, but can be heard on inspiration.

- CAUSED by air rushing past a constricted airway, constricted by secretions, mucous, edema, neurogenic, a tumour, or an aspirated foreign body.

- Asthma: Wheezing is characteristic of asthma.

    o **Silent Asthma** is asthma without wheezing.

- **STRIDOR:** High-pitched sound occurring with inspiration.

    o Strider portends total airway obstruction, a medical emergency.

- **Acute Epiglottitis:** H. Influenza infection in kids. Strider is characteristic. Have a chest-tube nearby before examining epiglottis to prevent (or treat imminent) aspiration.

CYANOSIS:

- Central Cyanosis: Face, lips, tongue. Results from systemic hypoxia due to poor perfusion or ventilation in the lungs.

- Peripheral Cyanosis: May be found in extremities, ears, cheeks, etc. Can be caused by cold-induced vasoconstriction (Raynaud's Phenomenon) or poor circulation (shock, CHF).

- Differential Diagnosis: Pulmonary hypoventilation, COPD

    o Cardiac causes: Shunt (Tetralogy of Fallot), pulmonary edema (cor pulmonale)

RHINORRHEA: Nasal discharge

- **CORYZA:** Nasal discharge caused by a viral upper respiratory tract infection.

FAMILY/ SOCIAL HISTORY:

- Previous Tuberculosis infection, PPD test.

- Poor dental hygiene is a risk for a lung abscess.

- Environmental exposures revealed in social history
    - Travel
    - Psittacosis: Exposure to birds
    - Legionellosis: Exposure to water, air-conditioners

- Tobacco use.

EXTRAPULMONARY EXAMINATION:

- **HALITOSIS:** Some possible causes:
    - Campylobacter Pylori colonization of stomach
    - Lung abscess or bronchiectasis (foul-smelling, fecal breath-odour)
    - Necrotic lesions of mouth or throat
    - Zenker's Diverticulum

- **CLUBBING OF FINGERNAILS**:
    - Congenital Heart Disease: Chronic hypoxia of VSD or Tetralogy, in kids.
    - Adults: Systemic hypoxia, lung cancer, bronchiectasis, **mesothelioma.**

- **CHEMOSIS:** Conjunctival edema. Hyperthyroidism or obstruction of SVC.

BREATHING:

- **BRADYPNEA:** Slow breathing rate
  - Insulin Coma
  - Drug-induced respiratory depression
- **TACHYPNEA:** Rapid, shallow breathing, caused by pleuritic chest pain or diseases that immobilize the lung.
- **HYPERPNEA:** Rapid, deep breathing; hyperventilation.
  - Diabetic ketoacidosis compensation (to lower PCO_2)
  - **KUSSMAUL RESPIRATIONS:** Central hyperventilation, deep rapid breaths characteristic of Diabetic hyperglycaemic coma.
- **CHEYNE-STOKES RESPIRATION:** Cyclic alternations between apnea and hyperpnea, in which PCO_2 fluctuates and is unstable. It occurs when the respiratory centres of the brain become insensitive to changes in CO_2.
  - ASSOCIATED DISEASES: Congestive Heart Failure (CHF), Uremia, Meningitis, Pneumonia.
- **BIOT'S BREATHING:** Ataxic breathing; unpredictable and irregular respirations.
  - Caused by meningitis or another cerebral dysfunction.
- **SLEEP APNEA:** Obesity, leading to airway obstruction at night and chronic fatigue during the day. Treat with CPAP.

INSPECTION:

BACK SIDE:

- **Buffalo Hump:** Fatty deposit overlying C7, characteristic of Cushing's Syndrome.

- **Barrel Chest:** Chronically inflated lungs characteristic of COPD.

- **Kyphosis:** Excessive anterior curvature of spine, as in hunchback.

    o   Causes: normal or from aging, **osteoporosis.**

- **Scoliosis:** Lateral curvature of spine.

    o   May be detected by patient bending forward and noting uneven paravertebral back muscles.

- **Lordosis:** Excessive posterior curvature of spine. Bowing of lumbar and cervical spines together.

- **Gibbus Deformity:** Sharp change of angle of spine instead of gradual change. Characteristic of Pott's Disease, or Vertebral Tuberculosis.

FRONT SIDE:

- **Pectus Carinatum (Pigeon Chest):** Sternum placed forward, increased anteroposterior chest measurement.

    o   Found in **Marfan's Syndrome, Rickets**

- **Pectus Excavatum (Funnel-Chest):** Lower end of sternum is depressed inward. May also be found in Marfan's Syndrome or Rickets.

- **Flail Chest:** Caused by multiple fractures of ribs. One side of chest moves paradoxically relative to the other side of the chest.

PALPATION: Assess chest excursion by placing fingers at costovertebral angle and having patient inhale.

- **SUBCUTANEOUS EMPHYSEMA:** Air in subcutaneous space. Can occur in tracheostomy patients, or people with ARDS who have an endotracheal tube.

- **OLIVER'S SIGN:** Tracheal tug when patient lifts his chin up.
    - Indicative of Aortic Aneurysm, pulling trachea downward by pressure of left main bronchus.
- **TACTILE FREMITUS:** Vibration on lungs when you have patient say "ninety-nine".
    - Increased fremitus is found with pulmonary consolidation in pneumonia.
    - Fremitus cannot be heard below the level of fluid in emphysema or pleural effusion, because the fluid stops the sound from being transmitted further.

PNEUMOTHORAX: Trachea will shift toward opposite side as the pneumothorax. The side of the pneumothorax acquires positive pressure, thus trachea deviates to the other side.

- **Tracheal Deviation:** Tracheal deviation can be caused by other things than pneumothorax.
    - **Pleural Effusion, Emphysema** may also cause trachea to deviate to the opposite side.
    - **Atelectasis** of lung may cause trachea to deviate toward same side as diseased lung.
- **Tension Pneumothorax:** Medical emergency in which air enters the pleural cavity and is trapped during expiration.
    - Intrathoracic pressure builds to values higher than atmospheric pressure, compresses the lung, and may displace the mediastinum and its structures toward the opposite side, with consequent

PERCUSSION:

- **Resonance:** Normal breath sound

- **Hyperresonance:** Increased resonance over thorax.

    o   May be found in Emphysema or Pneumothorax.

- **Tympany:** Percussion of gastric air-bubble or air-filled bowel. Increased resonance.

- **Dullness:** Decreased resonance, normally found over liver, spleen, and below lung.

    o   Causes: Emphysema, Pneumonia with consolidation, pleural effusion.

- **Flatness:** Extreme dullness with few or no ringing tones.

    o   Pleural effusion, massive pulmonary consolidations with tumour, pneumonia.

AUSCULTATION:

General Properties:

- Stethoscope Sounds: Use the bell side to listen to breath sounds.

    o   Press lightly: hear low-pitched sounds.

    o   Press hard: hear high-pitched sounds.

    - Tracheal Breath Sounds: Loud, harsh, high-pitched.

    - Bronchial Breath Sounds: Loud, high-pitched with air swishing past.

    - Bronchovesicular Sounds: Heard near branching of main bronchi, combination of bronchial and vesicular sounds.

    - Vesicular Sounds: Soft, low-pitched, airy, swishing, heard below the level of the bronchi.

- **CRACKLES (RALES, CREPITATIONS):** Soft, short, high-pitched fine sounds.
  - CAUSES: Congestive heart failure, bronchitis, pneumonia, pulmonary edema, bronchiectasis.

- **RHONCHUS:** Snoring sound, characteristic of asthma. It indicates fluid or mucus in airways.

- **WHEEZE:** On expiration, squeaking high-pitched sound, often audible to unaided ear.
  - Caused by air passing by obstructed airway.
  - Characteristic of asthma, but also found in emphysema, bronchitis.

- **PLEURAL FRICTION RUB:** Grating sound heard during breathing that stops when the breath is held. Caused by friction of visceral and parietal pleura.

- **PULMONARY CONSOLIDATION:** Occurs with late-stage lobar pneumonia.
  - **BRONCHOPHONY:** Increased transmission of sound to the lung periphery. Indicative of pulmonary consolidation.
  - **WHISPERED PECTORILOQUY:** Words being understood better when whispered. Also indicative of pulmonary consolidation.
  - **EGOPHONY:** "E" to "A" sound-changes. Indicative of pulmonary consolidation or pleural effusion.

- **HAMMAN'S SIGN:** Crunching, crackling sound over chest heard synchronous with the heartbeat. Occurs with **mediastinal emphysema** – air in the mediastinum.
  - CAUSES: Can follow thoracic surgery, trauma.
    - **Boerhaave's Syndrome:** Esophageal rupture causing air in mediastinum. Rare.

LUNG DISEASES:

- **ASTHMA**
- **ATELECTASIS:** Bronchial plug ------> decreased lung volume--> higher lung density ------> lung mass is pulled toward chest wall by negative pressure.

    o   Tracheal deviation toward affected side.
    o   crackles, maybe.
    o   no breath sounds.

- **BRONCHIECTASIS:** Chronic bronchial dilation.

    o   Caused by frequent pulmonary infections or pneumonia.

    o   Large amounts of sputum will be expectorated when patient lies prone hanging toward floor.

- **BRONCHITIS:** Acute (infectious) or chronic (smoker's)

- **BRONCHIOLITIS:** Common in infants and children.

- **LUNG CANCER**

- **COR PULMONALE**

- **CROUP:** Kids under 3 years old. Rapid, staccato coughs.
    o   Differential Diagnosis is between inflammatory Croup or Spasmodic Croup.

- **CYSTIC FIBROSIS**

- **PLEURAL EFFUSION:** Dullness on percussion. Decreased fremitus. Reduced breath sounds.

- **EMPHYSEMA**

- **EPIGLOTTITIS:** In kiddies, don't inspect the pharynx without a chest tube nearby.

- **PNEUMONIA**

3.0 CARDIAC

CARDIAC SYMPTOMS, HISTORY:

CHEST PAIN

ANGINA (ISCHEMIC CARDIAC PAIN): Squeezing, crushing, strangling, constricting pain in centre of chest. Pain may radiate to left shoulder, left arm, right shoulder, jaw.

- **Stable (typical) Angina:** Angina upon effort, or angina induced by increased blood pressure or increased heart-rate. Angina is relieved by nitroglycerin, although nitroglycerin is not specific to this type of angina.

    o Levine's Sign: Patient makes fist and holds it up to his chest, to describe the pain.

    o Second-wind Phenomenon: If patient repeats same activity after the attack, he may not feel the attack again the second time.

    o Walk-through Angina: The pain subsides as patient continues the activity.

- **Atypical Angina:** Atypical presentation of typical angina.

    o *Atypical Symptoms:* Sharp or stabbing pain, rather than crushing pain.

    o *Atypical Causes:* Angina with change in position, for example, rather than angina strictly upon effort.

    o *Angina Equivalents:* Other symptoms that are caused by myocardial ischemia.

    - Exertional dyspnea.

    - Nausea, indigestion.

    - Dizziness, sweating.

- **Unstable Angina:** Angina even at rest, or angina that has recently got worse. It is associated with sharply increased risk for myocardial infarct within 4 months.
    o **Angina Decubitus** is a specific term for angina occurring at rest.
- **Variant Angina (Prinzmetal Angina):** Paradoxical angina occurring during rest but usually not during exercise. It is caused by coronary artery spasm. It can be hard to spot because it can coexist with typical angina.
    o Characteristic ECG findings can help distinguish variant angina from typical angina.
    o Nitroglycerin will probably still relieve pain, as it relaxes coronary arteries.
- **Myocardial Infarct:** Typical presentation Unstable angina lasting longer than 15 minutes, that is not relieved by nitroglycerin.
    o Silent MI's and MI's with atypical presentation do occur.

NON-ISCHEMIC CARDIAC PAIN:
- **Mitral Valve Prolapse:** Usually asymptomatic, but may present with an intermittent, sharp, sticking pain over left precordium.
- **Pericarditis:** The patient feels relief by shallow breathing and by sitting up and leaning forward.
- **Dissecting Aneurysm:** Sudden, severe tearing pain, radiating to the abdomen, neck, or back, depending on where the aneurysm is going.

PLEURITIC (PULMONARY) CHEST PAIN: Also see pulmonary study guide.

- **Pulmonary Embolism:** May be asymptomatic, or the patient may feel a dull tightness if the embolus is large enough.
    o **Paroxysmal Dyspnea** is the most common symptom of pulmonary embolism.

- **Pleurisy:** Pain upon breathing. May be caused by pulmonary embolism, pneumonia, bronchitis, or pleural effusion.
- **Pulmonary Hypertension:** Dyspnea is a more common symptom than pleuritic pain.
- **Pneumothorax:** Pain may be confused with pain of an MI.
- **Mediastinal Emphysema:** Free air in the mediastinum produces chest tightness and dyspnea.
    - Hamman's Sign: Crunching, rasping sound heard synchronous with the heartbeat, indicative of mediastinal emphysema.

GASTROINTESTINAL CHEST PAIN:

- **Esophageal Spasm:** Substernal chest pain and dysphagia.
- **Esophageal Reflux (GERD):** Chest pain relieved by antacids.
- **Gallstone Colic:** Colicky RUQ pain radiating to back and to right shoulder. Occasionally it may be confused with angina.

CHEST WALL PAIN:

- **TIETZE'S SYNDROME (COSTOCHONDRITIS):** Inflammation of Costochondral joints. Pain is often localized and can be elicited by palpating the sternum over the involved ribs.
- **HERPES ZOSTER:** Pain may precede the appearance of the rash. Both pain and rash follow dermatomal distribution.
- **DACOSTA'S SYNDROME:** Psychogenic pain
- Usually localized to the cardiac apex. May be associated with anxiety.
    - May also see palpitations, hyperventilation, dyspnea, weakness, depression, or other signs of anxiety.
- **VERTEBRAL COLUMN DISEASE:** It may occasionally lead to anterior chest pain.

***DYSPNEA*:** Air hunger or difficulty breathing may be associated with cardiac diseases.

- **EXERTIONAL DYSPNEA:** Dyspnea on exertion is a common symptom of mild or severe Congestive Heart Failure.

- **DYSPNEA at REST:**

    o **Pulmonary** causes of dyspnea (PE, COPD, pneumothorax) often occur at rest. With cardiac problems, dyspnea usually does not occur at rest, or it is overshadowed by angina.

    o **Anxiety Dyspnea:** Difficulty breathing due to anxiety occurs only at rest.

- **ORTHOPNEA:** Dyspnea occurring with patient in the supine position. Orthopnea is a sign of **Congestive Heart Failure** that is more severe than that associated with exertional dyspnea.

    o CAUSE: Supine position increases pulmonary blood flow ------> exacerbate pulmonary congestion and pulmonary edema. The problem is relieved by resuming a more upright position.

    o Two-Pillow, Three-Pillow Orthopnea: Terms to describe the severity of the orthopnea. Three pillows are worse than two-pillow.

- **PAROXYSMAL NOCTURNAL DYSPNEA (PND):** Similar to orthopnea, except it has sudden onset and occurs only after the patient has been lying down at rest for at least an hour.

    o Unlike orthopnea, it is not relieved immediately by sitting up.

    o Patient is usually able to return to sleep, eventually.

- **PULMONARY EDEMA:** Pulmonary edema is usually a manifestation of left-ventricular heart failure. Peripheral edema associated with CHF is a manifestation of right-sided heart failure (Cor Pulmonale).

- o SYMPTOMS: Severe symptoms. Extreme anxiety, dyspnea, air hunger, cold sweats, fear of impending death.
- o SIGNS: Pink, frothy sputum, and bubbly breath sounds.

- **VALVULAR HEART DISEASE:** Mitral Stenosis is associated with dyspnea.
- **CONGENITAL HEART DISEASES:**
  - o Tetralogy of Fallot: Exertional dyspnea is common.

  - o Ventricular Septal Defect: Tachypnea and sweating. Late cyanosis.
- **CARDIAC -vs- PULMONARY DYSPNEA:**
- **OTHER CAUSES OF SHORTNESS OF BREATH:**
  - o **Kussmaul Respiration:** Intense hyperventilation (respiratory alkalosis) occurring with **Diabetic Ketoacidosis,** as a compensatory mechanism to relieve the metabolic acidosis.

PALPITATIONS: An unpleasant awareness of one's own heartbeat. Often described as fluttering, or skipping a beat.

- **PAROXYSMAL ATRIAL TACHYCARDIA:** May cause palpitations with an instantaneous onset.

- **PREMATURE VENTRICULAR CONTRACTIONS (PVC'S):** May be experienced as palpitations or a skipped beat. The premature contraction is followed by a compensatory pause, to allow for ventricular filling.

FATIGUE: Non-specific finding often found with heart disease.

- **FATIGUE CAUSED BY HEART DISEASE:** It usually occurs later in the day or in the evening. Fatigue early in the morning is usually not associated with heart disease, unless the patient was aroused from REM sleep.

  - o The heart disease gets worse, as the patient experiences onset of fatigue earlier in the day.

- **OTHER CAUSES OF FATIGUE:** Lots. Chronic illness of many types, anemia, psychological causes.

SYNCOPE: Fainting, transient loss of consciousness.

- **VASOVAGAL EVENTS:** Most common cause of syncope, it is caused by excessive stimulation of the Vagus nerve --> excessive bradycardia and reduced blood-flow to the brain.
    - **Anxiety:** It is usually associated with acute anxiety or excessive emotion. The Vagal hyperactivity is thought to be a hypersensitive response to sympathetic outflow.
- **CARDIOVASCULAR CAUSES:**
    - **Arrhythmias:**
        - **STOKES-ADAMS SYNDROME:** Syncope caused by reduced cardiac output secondary to an arrhythmia.
        - Both severe tachycardia and bradycardia can reduce cardiac output, leading to syncope. Severe tachycardia reduces cardiac output by reducing ventricular filling time.
    - **Cardiac Outflow Tract Obstruction:**
        - **Aortic Stenosis** may lead to syncope.
        - **Myxomas,** benign myocardial tumours, may cause outflow obstruction and lead to syncope.
        - **Tetralogy of Fallot** is associated with fainting attacks.
    - **Myocardial Ischemia**
    - **Carotid Sinus Syncope**: Hypersensitivity of the Carotid Sinus in elderly men is common cause of syncope.
    - **Impaired Vasomotor Reflexes:** Impairment of Baroreceptors. Syncope is associated with orthostatic hypotension.
    - **Decreased Blood Volume**

- **FLUID REMOVAL:**

    o **Micturition Syncope:** Syncope occurring with micturition but at no other time. Associated with removal of fluid from the body.

- **POST-TUSSIVE SYNCOPE:** Syncope after a bout of coughing, or after the Valsalva manoeuvre, may occur in patients with COPD.

HEMOPTYSIS: Mitral Valve Stenosis is a cardiac disease that may cause hemoptysis. Mitral Stenosis -----> pulmonary venous congestion ------> may lead to hemoptysis.

EDEMA:

- Pitting Edema is a common sign of Congestive Heart Failure.

- Presacral Edema may be found in bed-ridden patients, and may lead to decubitus ulcers.

- Anasarca: Severe generalized edema and ascites, as seen in severe CHF, liver cirrhosis, or nephrotic syndrome.

- Lymphedema may be caused Filariasis or a tumour obstructing a lymphatic vessel.

CYANOSIS: Presence of excessive deoxygenated hemoglobin in the blood. It becomes visible when the concentration of deoxygenated hemoglobin exceeds 5 g / dL – a higher rate of desaturation than is found in the venous blood of normal people.

- **Central Cyanosis:** Visible in the lips, face, conjunctivae, tongue. It is caused by primary systemic hypoxia due to impaired oxygenation of blood. EXAMPLES:
    o **Tetralogy of Fallot** or the late stages of other congenital heart defects
    o **Veno-arterial shunt**

- **Peripheral Cyanosis (Acrocyanosis):** Visible in the fingers and toes, earlobes, nose. It is caused by localized hypoxia due to poor circulation, reduced blood-flow, CHF, shock.

GENERAL PHYSICAL EXAM: Many congenital disorders are associated with various heart defects.

- THE FACE:
- THE EYES:
- THE MOUTH:
- THE SKIN:
    - **Rheumatic Fever:** Characteristically you will see **Erythema Marginatum** and Subcutaneous Nodules.

- THE THORAX:
- THE ABDOMEN:
- THE EXTREMITIES:
    - **Clubbing** of fingers and toes is a classic finding of **Cyanosis.** May also be seen with infective endocarditis or other conditions.

BLOOD PRESSURE:

- **PALPATION:**
- **AUSCULTATION (Korotkoff Sounds):**
    - **Phase 1:** Clear tapping sounds representing systolic pressure.
    - **Phase 2:** Softer tones
    - **Phase 3:** Louder once again.

- o **Phase 4:** Muffled Tones.

- o **Phase 5:** Tones cease. Diastolic Pressure. Diastolic pressure may actually be higher than estimated by auscultation.

- **INTERPRETATION:**

  - o Auscultatory Gap: Period of silence that may occur between Phase 1 and Phase 2. The beginning and end of the Auscultatory Gap may be mistaken for Diastolic or Systolic blood pressure, respectively.
    - CAUSES: Venous distension or severe Aortic Stenosis.
  - o **Orthostatic Hypotension:** Upon standing, normal decrease in systolic blood pressure is 5-15 mm Hg; anything more is Orthostatic Hypotension. Diastolic pressure normally remains constant or increases slightly.
  - o Obese Patient: Use a large cuff.
  - o Hypertension:
    - Coarctation of the Aorta will result in a systolic pressure that is quite high in the arm, but much lower in the leg.

JUGULAR VENOUS PULSES:

- **Central Venous Pressure (CVP):** Use the right Internal Jugular to estimate CVP because it is straighter.

  - o MEASUREMENT:

    - With patient sitting up, clavicles are 10 cm above right atrium, thus CVP = jugular venous distension above clavicles + 10 cm.

    - With patient elevated 30, sternal Angle of Louis is normally about 5 cm above right atrium, and Internal Jugular should be visible about 3 cm directly vertical (use a ruler), above the sternal Angle of Louis.

- o RESPIRATION: CVP should decrease with inspiration and increase with expiration.

    - KUSSMAUL'S SIGN: Paradoxical change in CVP during inspiration (and increase instead of decrease), caused by a restriction in filling of the right ventricle, such as pericardial effusion.

    - HEPATOJUGULAR REFLEX: Normally, it should only show a transient increase in CVP. With Cor Pulmonale, the increased CVP is maintained throughout.

- **JUGULAR VENOUS WAVES:**

  - o **a-Wave:** Right atrial contraction, corresponding to peak filling of the jugular vein.

    - A large a-wave is characteristic of pulmonary hypertension.

    - A giant a-wave is characteristic of a total heart block.

    - No a-wave is characteristic of atrial fibrillation.

  - o **x-Descent:** Follows a-wave, as atrium relaxes. Decreased jugular vein filling.

    - First heart sound is heard during the

  - o **c-Wave:** Occurs with contraction of the ventricles. Usually not visible at bedside.

    - CAROTID PULSE occurs during this, which is right after the a-wave and also during the x-descent.

  - o **v-Wave:** Passive phase of atrial filling during ventricular systole.

  - o **y-Descent:** Brief decreases in jugular vein pressure after the Tricuspid valve opens (beginning of Systole).

ARTERIAL PULSES:

- **NORMAL PULSES**: Radial, Brachial, Carotid, Femoral, Popliteal, Posterior Tibial, Dorsalis Pedis.

- **RHYTHM ABNORMALITIES:**

    o **Sinus Arrhythmia:** The pulse accelerates with inspiration.

    o Premature Contractions:

    - **Atrial Premature Contractions (APC):** Normally do not disturb the cycle.

    - **Ventricular Premature Contractions (PVC):** They are followed by a compensatory pause, and a new rhythm is established.

    o **Pulse Deficit:** With **Atrial Fibrillation + Tachycardia,** the radial pulse may not be equal to the cardiac apical pulse. Two rapid beats in a row may not allow sufficient ventricular filling for the systole to be transmitted to the periphery. The lapse between apical and radial pulse is the pulse deficit.

    o **Bigeminal Pulse:** Two consecutive heartbeats closely coupled, with subsequent pause before the next beat.

- **VOLUME ABNORMALITIES:**

    o **Hyperkinetic Pulse:** Quick up stroke and full volume, seen with hypertension, anxiety.

    o **Corrigan's Pulse:** A brisk pulse with large volume, or "Collapsing" pulse, seen in Aortic Regurgitation.

    - **Duroziez Murmur** should be heard across the femoral artery simultaneous with the collapsing pulse.

    o **Quincke's Pulse:** Visible capillary pulsations in the nail-bed. Another sign of Aortic Insufficiency.

- **Pulsus Bisferiens:** Bifid pulse. Two distinct impulses with each heartbeat. Seen in:

    - Aortic Regurgitation

    - Hypertrophic Cardiomyopathy.

- **Pulsus Alterans:** One pulse feels large, the next one small. Due to decreased cardiac contractility and carries a poor prognosis.

- **Pulsus Paradoxus:** Weakening of the pulse with inspiration more than normal.

    - Systolic pressure normally decreases by less than 10 mm Hg. Paradoxical pulse occurs when decrease is greater than 10 mm Hg.

    - Indicative of constrictive cardiac disease: Pericardial effusion, constrictive pericarditis.

- Grading Pulses: Scale of 0 to 4

  - Scale:

    - **0** = no pulse

    - **3** = normal pulse

    - **4** = bounding pulse

  - **Intermittent Claudication:** Temporary weakening of lower extremities due to arterial insufficiency.

  - **Leriche's Syndrome:** Atherosclerosis of abdominal Aorta, reducing flow to lower extremities and leading to impotence.

  - **Takayasu's Disease:** Pulseless disease – no pulse in arms, due to progressive obliterative arteritis.

THE PRECORDIUM:

- **AORTIC VALVE:** Second right interspace (upper right – on the opposite side because the Aorta bends over toward the right side).

- **PULMONIC VALVE:** Second left interspace (upper left – on opposite side because the Pulmonary arteries bifurcate behind the Aorta).

- **TRICUSPID VALVE:** Lower parasternum (centrally located).

- **MITRAL VALVE:** Apex

- **ERB'S POINT:** Place to listen to right-sided pathologies, at the third left interspace.

PALPATION / PERCUSSION:

- **POINT OF MAXIMAL IMPULSE (PMI):** Should be at the apex.

    - If it is located more centrally and down, that is indicative of **COPD** due to barrel chest and constantly inflated lungs, displacing the heart centrally (right-sided shift).

    - Right Ventricular Hypertrophy can shift the PMI posteriorly, as the right-ventricular mass masks the left-ventricular PMI, making it difficult to palpate.

- **SHOCK:** An impulse of a heart sound transmitted to the examining hand.

- **HEAVE / LIFT:** Forceful, systolic thrust that moves the palpating hand up a little.

- **THRILL:** A palpable murmur. A palpable vibration that by definition is accompanied by an audible murmur.

***STETHOSCOPE*:** Get a good one. The shorter the tube, the better. Double-barrelled tubes are better than single barrel.

- **DIAPHRAGM:** High-pitched (primarily systolic) sounds and press firmly.

- **BELL:** Low-pitched (primarily diastolic) sounds and press lightly.

HEART SOUNDS:

- **NORMAL HEART SOUNDS:** Normal order of events = **M1, T1, A2, P2**

    o **S1:** Closing of Mitral (M1) and Tricuspid (T1) valves.

    - 51 is loudest near the apex.

    - LOUD 51: Occurs with higher cardiac output, such as fever, exercise, thyrotoxicosis.

    - SOFT 51: Occurs with impaired myocardial.

    - contraction, CHF, mitral regurgitation.

    o **S2:** Closing of Aortic (A2) and Pulmonic (P2) valves.

    - SPLITTING: Normally, Aortic closes before Pu/manic,

    - due to higher pressure in Aorta.
        - **Wide Splitting:** INSPIRATION normally increases the interval between A2 and P2, which is attributed to increased pulmonary blood flow, and decreased pulmonary vascular resistance.

    - INTENSITY: A loud S2 usually is attributed to the Aortic valve (A2), and often occurs with hypertension.

- **THIRD HEART SOUND (S3):** Considered normal in infants and children.

    o CAUSE: Slowing of velocity of blood, or vibrations from turbulent blood-flow during ventricular filling, especially at the beginning.

    o POSITION: Patient should be in left lateral decubitus position for maximal auscultation of S3.

    o **Gallop:** S3 sound plus tachycardia, giving the sound of a galloping horse.

    o ETIOLOGIES: Cardiac disease which causes increased ventricular volume, such as:

        - Mitral and Tricuspid Regurgitation
        - Congestive Heart Failure

    o **Opening Snap (OS):** Brief click heard when mitral valve opens at the beginning of diastole (around S3). Associated with Mitral Stenosis

    o **Kentucky:** Sl, S2, S3 together have this approximate rhythm.

- **FOURTH HEART SOUND (S4):** Always pathological.

    o CAUSE: Contraction of the atria at the end of diastole --> turbulent blood flow which is audible as S4.

        - Decreased ventricular compliance is the most common etiology of S4 sound.

    o ETIOLOGIES:

        - Left-Sided: hypertension, aortic stenosis, angina pectoris.
        - Right Sided: pulmonary hypertension, pulmonic stenosis.

- o **Tennessee:** 54, 51, 52 sounds together have this approximate rhythm.

- **SUMMATION GALLOP:** S3 + S4 + Tachycardia, as seen in chronic hypertension leading to CHF.

- **SYSTOLIC SOUNDS and CLICKS:**

  - o Ejection Sounds: Can be innocent or caused by abnormal Aortic valves or a dilated Aorta.

  - o Mitral Valve Prolapse (MVP): Will result in a mid or late systolic click, as the mitral leaflet protrudes back into the atrium during ventricular contraction.

- **NON-VALVULAR SOUNDS:**

  - o **Precordial Knock:** Results from **constrictive pericarditis** and can be heard over the internal jugular at the base of the neck.

    - CAUSE: thickened pericardium limits expansion of ventricles during rapid filling phase of diastole, resulting in backup of blood.

  - o **Pericardial Friction Rub:** Caused by **pericardial effusion** and can be heard over a limited area in left parasternal space.

    - More extensive pericardial effusion may eliminate the rub, as the pericardium gets completely separated from the epicardium.

HEART MURMURS: General Properties

- **TIMING**

- **LOCATION**

- **CONFIGURATION: CRESCENDO/ DECRESCENDO**

- **INTENSITY:**
  - **Grade I:** Barely audible by an expert.
  - **Grade III:** Moderately loud with palpable thrill.
  - **Grade VI:** So loud it can be heard without the stethoscope making complete contact with the skin.
- **FREQUENCY**
- **QUALITY**
- **TRANSMISSION**: Where does the sound transmit to? This is characteristic for certain pathologies and can be diagnostic.

SYSTOLIC MURMURS: Cardiac disorders and their associated findings.

- **AORTIC STENOSIS:** Diamond-shaped systolic ejection murmur.
  - Location: Over the Aortic valve, at the second right intercostal space.
  - Transmission: to the carotids bilaterally.
- **PULMONIC STENOSIS:** Diamond-shaped systolic ejection murmur.
  - Location: Second or third left parasternal interspace.
- **HYPERTROPHIC OBSTRUCTIVE CARDIOMYOPATHY:** *Diamond-shaped midsystolic murmur.*
  - PATHOLOGY of DISEASE:
    - Septal region of left ventricle is thickened > Left Ventricular Hypertrophy.

- During systole, anterior leaflet of mitral valve is abnormal.
- Impaired relaxation of the left ventricle during diastole.

  o SOUND: Similar to Aortic Stenosis, but it does not transmit to the Carotids.

  o EXAMINATION TECHNIQUES: The murmur becomes louder as left ventricular volume is reduced. This is paradoxic behaviour as compared to most murmurs
    - **Handgrip** ------> increase in left ventricular volume ------> decreased murmur. This occurs because the septa! obstruction is relatively less significant.
    - **Valsalva Maneuver:** Murmur becomes louder in the late-stage of the Valsalva Maneuver, rather than softer as in most murmurs.
    - Murmur becomes quieter when the patient squats – also paradoxical behaviour.

- **MITRAL VALVE PROLAPSE:** If it occurs with mitral regurgitation, a late systolic murmur will be heard after the midsystolic click.

  o Examination Technique: Like cardiomyopathy, reduce left ventricular volume ------> louder murmur (and an earlier click).

- **HOLOSYSTOLIC MURMURS:** They indicate that blood is flowing down a pressure gradient when it shouldn't be, as in insufficiencies.

  o CAUSES: Mitral regurgitation, Tricuspid regurgitation, Ventricular septal defect.

- **MITRAL REGURGITATION:** The most common cause for *Holosystolic Murmur.*

  o Causes: Anything that makes the mitral valve incompetent, or mitral leaflets damage:

- Vegetations
- papillary muscle dysfunction
- shortened chordae tendineae

  o Concurrent features of Mitral Regurgitation:
  - Left Ventricular Hypertrophy ------> Shifted PMI
  - S3 gallop

- **VENTRICULAR SEPTAL DEFECT:** Best heard at lower left parasternal border (Erb's point)
- **TRICUSPID REGURGITATION:** Holosystolic murmur

  o May result from IV drug use ------> endocarditis, or Rheumatic valvular disease.

- **OTHER MURMURS:**

  o **STRAIGHT BACK SYNDROME:** Systolic ejection murmur.
  o **Innocent Murmurs**
  o **Venous Hum:** Heard above the clavicles in normal individuals.
  o **Mammary Souffle:** High-pitched continuous flow heard over base of heart in pregnancy.

DIASTOLIC MURMURS: Cardiac disorders and associated findings.

- **AORTIC INSUFFICIENCY:** Blowing or Decrescendo diastolic murmur.

  o Many causes: infectious, rheumatic, dissecting aortic aneurysm.
  o CHF makes the murmur softer.
  o Associated findings:

- **Corrigan's Water Hammer Pulse:** Collapsing pulse, with little up stroke or downstroke.
- de Musset's Sign: to and fro head movement synchronous with the heartbeat.
- **Quincke's Pulse:** capillary pulsation of fingertips.
- **Duroziez's Sign:** Femoral artery systolic and diastolic bruits.
- **Hill's Sign:** Blood pressure in the legs being higher than it is in the arms.
  - Normal difference = 20 mm Hg
  - Aortic Insufficiency = 40-60 mm Hg.

- **PULMONIC INSUFFICIENCY:** Decrescendo diastolic murmur.

  o **GRAHAM STEELL'S MURMUR: Pulmonary Hypertension** as the cause of pulmonic hypertension (due to dilation of pulmonic leaflets).

   - Prominent a-wave is found concurrent with the murmur.
   - Paradoxical Splitting also occurs.

- **MITRAL STENOSIS:** Middiastolic murmur

  o CAUSE: Chronic **Rheumatic Heart Disease** is most common cause.

- **TRI CUSPID STENOSIS:** *Middiastolic murmur*

- **RHEUMATIC FEVER:**

  o **Carey Coombs Murmur** is the characteristic murmur occurring during the acute stage of Rheumatic Fever. It is a blubbering Middiastolic murmur heard at apex. The murmur disappears after acute disease has subsided.

  o Middiastolic murmur of mitral stenosis might then remain as a sequel.

- **PATENT DUCTUS ARTERIOSUS:**

    o **Continuous Murmurs:** Murmurs occurring throughout the cardiac cycle, caused by blood continually flowing from higher pressure to lower pressure.

TECHNIQUES FOR ENHANCING AUSCULTATION:

- **INSPIRATION:** Normally you should see splitting of S2 with inspiration. P2 occurs later and moves further away from A2.

    o **Paradoxical Splitting:** S2 splitting is decreased instead of increased with inspiration.

    - **Left Bundle-Branch Block** causes paradoxical splitting. In this condition, under normal circumstances, A2 already occurs after P2 (instead of before), because of the left-sided heart-block. Thus, with inspiration, P2 actually moves closer to A2 and you see paradoxical splitting.

- **EXHALATION:** Can be used to evaluate right-sided heart murmurs.

    o The intensity of most right-sided heart murmurs will decrease with exhalation, while left-sided murmurs remain unchanged.

- **MULLER'S MANEUVER:** Have patient pinch the nostrils shut with one hand and suck hard on a finger with the other.

    o MECHANISM: This creates prolonged **negative intrathoracic pressure.** That shift blood from the systemic to the pulmonary circulation, which amplifies and prolongs the murmurs found with inspiration. It makes it easier to hear inspiratory murmurs.

- **VALSALVA MANEUVER:** Have patient hold breath and bear down for 20 seconds. Can be used to evaluate left-sided heart murmurs.

    o MECHANISM: This creates a prolonged **positive**

intrathoracic pressure. That shifts blood from the pulmonary to the systemic circulation – the exact opposite as Muller's Maneuver.

- o TIME COURSE: Most left-side murmurs first grow louder, and then grow softer.

- o First 10-15 seconds: Initially, cardiac output increases, and the intensity of left-sided murmurs increase accordingly.

- o After 10-15 seconds: Cardiac then begins to decrease, as venous return from the lungs decreases. Most left-sided murmurs then grow softer again.

- **EXCEPTIONS:** Two conditions show different characteristics than above:

  - o **Hypertrophic Obstructive Cardiomyopathy:** Left-ventricular hypertrophy and resultant cardiomyopathy, due to hypertension. With this condition, the late phase of the murmur actually increases or may be heard for the first time.

  - o **Mitral Valve Prolapse:** Late-phase murmur usually increases rather than decreases and may be heard for the first time.

- **STANDING to SQUATTING:** Have patient squat down and breathe normally, and then stand. Squatting increases stroke volume and standing decreases it again.

  - o **Hypertrophic Obstructive Cardiomyopathy:** As patient squats, this murmur should be decreased.

  - o **Mitral Regurgitation:** Occasionally decreases.

- **SQUATTING to STANDING:**

  - o **Hypertrophic Obstructive Cardiomyopathy:** As the patient stands back, this murmur should increase.

  - o **Mitral Regurgitation:** Occasionally increases.

- **PASSIVE LEG ELEVATION:**

  o **Hypertrophic Obstructive Cardiomyopathy:**

  o Murmur should decrease, as left ventricular volume increases and the left ventricle enlarges.

- **ISOMETRIC HANDGRIP:** Using a handgrip for 1 minute increases peripheral vascular resistance.

  o DECREASED INTENSITY: Hypertrophic Obstructive Cardiomyopathy, Aortic Stenosis (about 30% of cases).

  o INCREASED INTENSITY: Ventricular Septal Defect, Aortic Regurgitation, Mitral Regurgitation.

  o CONTRAINDICATIONS: Do not do this test on people with myocardial ischemia, ventricular arrhythmias, or unstable angina

- **TRANSIENT ARTERIAL OCCLUSION:** Place blood pressure cuff on both arms and occlude blood-flow for 20 seconds.

  o INCREASED INTENSITY: Mitral Regurgitation, Ventricular Septal Defect. Most other murmurs are unaffected.

- **AMYL NITRATE:** Have patient inhale amyl nitrate > decreased TPR. Auscultate sounds 15-30 seconds later.

  o DECREASED INTENSITY: Mitral Regurgitation, Ventricular Septal Defect.

  o INCREASED INTENSITY: Right-sided murmurs, aortic stenosis, hypertrophic obstructive cardiomyopathy.

4.0 ABDOMEN

HISTORY TAKING:

ABDOMINAL PAIN

- **CHARACTER OF PAIN**
    - **PUD:** Burning or gnawing pain, epigastric, may radiate to the back.
        - Precipitated by long periods of no food or skipping meals.
        - Often feel pain early in morning, which is relieved by intake of food or antacids.
    - **GERD:** Burning, epigastric or xiphisternal. Radiates to the retrosternum.
        - Precipitated by over-eating, bending over, or being in a reclined position.

- **LOCATION OF PAIN:**

- **RADIATION OF PAIN**
    - **Renal Colic often radiates to the groin.**
    - **Gallbladder pain often radiates to back, scapula, or right shoulder.**
    - **Splenic pain often radiates to back.**
    - **Pancreatic pain often radiates to back.**

- **FACTORS PRECIPITATING AND RELIEVING THE PAIN**

- **PATIENT ASSESSMENT OF PAIN SEVERITY:** Scale of 0 to 10.

- **COMPARISON WITH OTHER TYPES OF PAIN**

ANOREXIA:

- **DIFFERENTIAL DIAGNOSIS:**
  - Neoplasms
  - Chronic Renal Failure
  - Psychiatric: Anorexia nervosa, depression
  - Infections: Hepatitis, many chronic infections.
- **POLYPHAGIA**: Seen in hyperthyroidism, malabsorption syndromes, especially pancreatic insufficiency.

NAUSEA AND VOMITING:

- **DELAYED GASTRIC EMPTYING:** It is a common cause of nausea. Possible causes of delayed gastric emptying:
  - Pyloric Outlet Obstruction: Ulcers, pyloric stenosis, Crohn's Disease, neoplasms.
  - Neuromuscular: Scleroderma, vagotomy, demyelinating diseases (MS), Polio.
  - Metabolic: **Diabetic gastroparesis, hypothyroidism.**
  - Drugs: Anti-cholinergics, ganglionic blockers, opiates.
  - Psychiatric: Anorexia Nervosa.
- **PROJECTILE VOMITING:** Special vomiting that can signify increased intracranial pressure (ICP).
- **REGURGITATION:** Vomiting without nausea. Causes:
  - Overeating.
  - Achalasia.
  - Delayed gastric emptying
  - Esophageal rings and webs.

DYSPHAGIA:

- **ODNYOPHAGIA:** Painful difficulty swallowing.
- Common Causes:
  - **VA, stroke**
  - Parkinson's
  - Reflux Esophagitis
  - Esophageal rings and webs
  - Achalasia
  - Esophageal Tumours
  - Candidiasis

DIARRHEA: Excretion of more than 300 g of stool per day.

- **ACUTE DIARRHEA:**
  - Infectious Gastroenteritis: Shigella, Salmonella, Campylobacter, invasive E. Coli.
    - Symptom Cluster: Fever, myalgia, chills, nausea, vomiting, diarrhea, cramping abdominal pain.
  - Lactose Intolerance
  - Antibiotic-associated (loss of normal flora)
  - Inflammatory bowel
- **STOOL INCONTINENCE:** Recurrent defecation in pants is not diarrhea and has a very limited differential diagnosis, all relating to anal sphincter dysfunction:
  - Diabetes Mellitus
  - Previous rectal or perirectal surgery.
  - Errant episiotomy from a traumatic childbirth.

- **CHRONIC DIARRHEA:**
    - Dietary habits (coffee).
    - Parasitic infection: giardiasis, amebiasis.
    - Inflammatory bowel disease.

CONSTIPATION: 2 bowel movements per week is normal in some people.

- **ACUTE CONSTIPATION:** Recent change in bowel habits. Causes:
    - Drugs: anticholinergics, psycho-active drugs, many others.
    - **Hypothyroidism**
    - **Hyperparathyroidism**
    - Decreased food intake, decreased fluid intake.
    - Chronic debilitating disease (post-stroke).

- **HIRSCHSPRUNG'S DISEASE:** Aganglionic Megacolon
    - Lifelong constipation
    - Occasional passage of enormous stools
    - Absence or marked diminution of ganglion cells in rectal tissue
    - Marked colonic distension.

- **IDIOPATHIC CHRONIC CONSTIPATION:** may be caused by a defect in the pelvis floor in women, in which they contract the anal sphincter, rather than relax it, when defecating

HEMATEMESIS

- Possible Causes:

    o   PUD or erosive Gastritis

    o   Mallory-Weiss Tear of esophagus

    o   Esophageal varices, portal hypertension

HEMATOCHEZIA and MELENA

- **HEMATOCHEZIA:** Occult blood in stool.

    o   Possible Causes
    o   **Colorectal carcinoma**
    o   **Infectious enteritis:** Shigella, Salmonella, Campylobacter, invasive E. Coli may all cause hematochezia.
    o   Hemorrhoids
    o   Chronic diverticular disease

- **MELENA:** Passage of black or very dark stool, reflecting heme breakdown products in stool.

    o   Other causes of black stool (other than occult blood): Iron-containing drugs, bismuth-containing drugs, charcoal, lots of black cherries.

- **MAROON-COLOURED STOOLS** are indicative of massive blood loss (2 to 3 units of blood). Usually, will see unstable vital signs. Look for complications of PUD, such as perforated ulcer.

INSPECTION:

PROTUBERANT OR DISTENDED ABDOMEN

- **PARTIAL BOWEL OBSTRUCTION:** Distended abdomen plus peristaltic movements heard over the distension is practically diagnostic.

- **PSEUDOCYESIS, PSEUDOPREGNANCY:** Woman who wants to be pregnant develops a distended abdomen psychogenically.

- Increased air in bowel causing abdominal distension:

    o Mechanical factors, carcinoma or adhesions

    o Adynamic paralytic ileus.

- **ASCITES:** Most common cause is alcoholic cirrhosis leading to portal hypertension.

    o **Fluid Wave:** Press down abdomen and create a fluid wave. It is indicative of ascites.

    o **Puddle Sign:** Have patient lie prone and then get on hands and knees, to get all ascites to go to a dependent position. Then flick and auscultate the abdomen, listening for changes in intensity of sounds. Positive test indicates ascites.

    o **Chylous Ascites** is milky (lipid) look to transudate, indicating lymphatic blockage. Occurs with intraabdominal lymphomas and Hodgkin's disease.

    o Ascites can be assessed by auscultation by assessing shifting dullness when patient changes position.

GREY TURNER'S SIGN: Ecchymoses on the abdomen, an unusual place for ecchymoses. It occurs in **fulminant acute pancreatitis** and carries a grave prognosis.

JAUNDICE:

- Most Common Causes
    o **Viral Hepatitis**
    o **Alcoholic Liver Disease**
    o **Drug-Induced Jaundice**
    o **Chronic Active Liver Disease**

- Choledocolithiasis
- Pancreatic Carcinoma
- Metastatic Liver Disease

ABDOMINAL HERNIAS:

- **ANATOMICAL TYPES OF HERNIAS:**

    - **Inguinal Hernias:** Most common hernia.

        - **Direct Inguinal Hernia:** Hernia directly penetrates the inguinal triangle. It creates a bulge right above (superior and medial to) the inguinal ligament.

        - **Indirect Inguinal Hernia:** Hernia passes through the inguinal canal, and creates a bulge in the right over the inguinal ligament, as it passes through the inguinal ring.
            - In men, often herniates into scrotum.

    - **Femoral Hernia:** Second most common. High risk of strangulation, 20% of cases.

    - **Obturator Hernia:** Unusual, occurring in elderly, thin, emaciated women. Protrusion of peritoneal sac through Obturator Foramen.

        - Symptom: Pain, paresthesia down anterior thigh, due to compression of femoral nerve.
    - **Umbilical Hernia:** May occur in people with chronic increased intraabdominal pressure: Multiparous women and COPD.
    - **Spigelian Hernia:** Occurs between umbilicus and pubic symphysis. Unusual.

- **REDUCIBILITY:**
    - **Reducible:** The contents of the hernia can be easily displaced.

- o **Irreducible, incarcerated:** The contents of the hernia cannot be displaced and are stuck there.

- o **Strangulated:** An incarcerated hernia that has cut off its blood supply, resulting in tissue necrosis and gangrene.

PERCUSSION:

- **TYMPANY:** Increased tympany is heard upon percussion of the abdomen in cases of **partial bowel obstruction.**

- **NORMAL LIVER SPAN:** 10-12 cm in men, 8-11 cm in women.

AUSCULTATION:

- **PERISTALTIC SOUNDS:**

    - o Absent Bowel Sounds: Ileus.

    - o Increased Bowel Sounds: Gastroenteritis.

    - o **Borborygmi:** High-pitched bowel sounds indicating small bowel obstruction.

- **SUCCUSSION SPLASH:** Audible presence of increased amount of fluid in stomach.

    - o Normal after a large meal.

    - o If it occurs after fasting, then it is indicative of **pyloric obstruction.**

- **ABDOMINAL BRUITS:** Caused by calcification of aorta, celiac compression, and alcoholic hepatitis.

- **PERITONEAL FRICTION RUBS:** Hearing a peritoneal friction rub over the liver is indicative of liver metastasis or primary hepatoma.

PALPATION:

LIVER:

- **HEPATOMEGALY:**
  - Primary or metastatic Hepatoma.
  - Alcoholic liver disease (fatty liver).
  - Severe CHF.
  - Infiltrative diseases of liver like amyloidosis.
  - Myeloproliferative Disorders: CML, Myelofibrosis.

SPLEEN

- **SPLENOMEGALY:**
  - **Infections**
  - **Leukemias**
  - **Portal hypertension**

GALLBLADDER

- **COURVOISIER'S LAW:** Gallbladder is palpable in 25% of cases of **pancreatic carcinoma**, due to painless distension.

- **Murphey's Sign:** RUQ pain aggravated by inspiration, indicative of **acute cholecystitis.**

KIDNEYS:

- **ENLARGED KIDNEYS:** Polycystic Kidney Disease, hypernephroma, renal cysts, hydronephrosis.

- **PTOTIC KIDNEY:** Normal-sized kidney displaced inferiorly into abnormal position; pelvic kidney.

AORTA: Pulsatile mass in midline is suggestive of Aortic Aneurysm.

MASSES and BOWEL LOOPS

FEMORAL PULSES and DISTAL AORTA: Decreased or absence femoral pulses can be found in several disorders

- **DISSECTING AORTIC ANEURYSM**
- **COARCTATION OF AORTA**
- **SEVERE ATHEROSCLEROTIC PERIPHERAL VASCULAR DISEASE**
- **LERICHE'S SYNDROME:** Occlusion of the distal Aorta.
  - Symptom Tetrad: Absent femoral pulses, intermittent claudication, gluteal pain, impotence.

RECTAL EXAM:

ACUTE ABDOMINAL PAIN:

LOCALIZING PAIN to INTRAABDOMINAL SITES. INVOLUNTARY GUARDING AND MUSCLE RIGIDITY:

- **PERFORATED ULCER**
- **PERFORATED BOWEL**
- **PERITONITIS**

DIRECT AND INDIRECT TENDERNESS

- **REBOUND TENDERNESS:** Tenderness on sudden release of pressure. A reliable sign of peritoneal inflammation.
- **JAR TENDERNESS:** Avoidance of sudden movements due to abdominal pain. Also, a sign of peritoneal inflammation.

ABDOMINAL PAIN SYNDROMES:

ACUTE ABDOMINAL PAIN

- **DIFFERENTIAL DIAGNOSIS:**
    - Infectious: Appendicitis, cholecystitis, pancreatitis, hepatitis, Gastroenteritis, Diverticulitis.
    - Crohn's Disease
    - **Bowel perforation:** Peritoneal signs should be present. Patient doesn't want to move.
    - **Bowel obstruction:** Patient can't stay still and keeps moving around to get comfortable.
    - Colic: Renal or biliary colic.
    - Dissecting Abdominal Aortic Aneurysm.
- **DIABETIC KETOACIDOSIS** and other metabolic disorders can simulate an acute abdomen.

CHRONIC ABDOMINAL PAIN:

- **PEPTIC ULCER DISEASE:** Gnawing, burning, aching.
    - Pain partially relieved by eating food.
    - Chronicity, Rhythmicity, Periodicity.

- **CHOLELITHIASIS and BILIARY COLIC:**
    - Paroxysms of sharp colicky RUQ pain, often radiating to back, right mid-abdomen.
    - Intolerance to greasy foods may be found.
    - Ultrasound is usually diagnostic.

- **DELAYED GASTRIC EMPTYING:**
    - Often accompanied by nausea, emesis, and early satiety.
    - Pain is worsened by eating.

- **CHRONIC PANCREATITIS:**
    - Caused by alcoholism.
    - May be exacerbated by eating.

- **PANCREATIC CARCINOMA**
    - Weight loss, abdominal pain, anorexia, weakness/ fatigue, diarrhea common.
    - Pain is variable in quality, and often ameliorated by sitting in knee-chest position.

- **LACTASE DEFICIENCY**

- **IRRITABLE BOWEL SYNDROME:** Abdominal discomfort with no demonstrable organic cause.
    - Defecation relieves the pain.

ANTERIOR ABDOMINAL WALL PAIN

- **NEUROMAS, HERPES ZOSTER, HERNIAS.**

- Tightening of abdominal wall should aggravate symptoms, indicating abdominal-wall pain. If tightening of abdominal wall relieved symptoms or were done as a guarding action, then that would be visceral pain.

5.0 MALE GENITALIA

SYMPTOMS:

- **DYSURIA:** Uncomfortable or painful urination

    o   Pain with urination: Urethritis, urethral obstruction, prostatitis.

    o   Pain felt after urination: **bladder calculus,** prostatitis.

- **FREQUENCY of URINATION:**

- **URGENCY:**

- **NOCTURIA:**

- **POLYURIA:**

- **URINARY INCONTINENCE:**

- **HEMATURIA:**

    o   **Time of Hematuria:**
    - Beginning of micturition: urethral or prostatic source. Blood is originating near the meatus.
    - Throughout micturition: renal source. Blood is diffusely present in urine.
    - End of micturition: bladder source. Blood is originating from bladder.

    o   **Painless Hematuria:** Think **neoplasms** (renal or bladder), renal tuberculosis, acute glomerulo-nephritis.

- **OLIGURIA, ANURIA:** Renal failure.

    o   **Oliguria:** 24-hr urine output less than 400 ml

    o   **Anuria:** 24-hr urine output less than 100 ml

- **PNEUMATURIA:** Passage of air or stool through urinary tract. It indicates the presence of fistula tracts connecting the GI and UG tracts, such as after surgery or with inflammatory bowel disease.

- **PROSTATISM:** No direct relationship exists between voiding habits and feelings of urgency, and the size of Benign Prostatic Hyperplasia.

- **PENILE PAIN, ULCERS, DISCHARGE:**
  - **Phimosis:** Constriction of the penis, causing pain in uncircumcised penises.

- **LOSS of LIBIDO, IMPOTENCE:**

- **INFERTILITY:**

- **SCROTAL SWELLING, TESTICULAR PAIN:** Testicular pain is usually caused by torsion, hydrocele, varicocele, or spermatocele. Testicular tumours are usually painless when they present.

PHYSICAL EXAM:

PENIS

- **BALANITIS:** Inflammation of the glans penis. Causes:
  - Diabetes mellitus
  - Infections: Candida, Trichomonas
  - Drug reactions
  - Reiter's Syndrome
- **PEYRONIE'S DISEASE**: Lateral deviation of penis, caused by unilateral inflammation of a corpus cavernosum.

SCROTUM

- **ATROPHIC TESTES:** Caused by orchitis, trauma, chronic **alcoholism, cirrhosis.**

- **HYDROCELE: Transillumination** of a scrotal mass will illuminate a hydrocele. If a painful mass is present, transilluminate it.

PROSTATE:

INGUINAL CANALS and GROIN: See abdominal study guide.

RECTAL EXAM:

6.0 FEMALE GENITALIA

SYMPTOMS

PAST HISTORY:

- **GRAVIDA:** Number of pregnancies

- **PARA:** Number of live deliveries

- Number of planned and spontaneous abortions

ABNORMALITIES in MENSTRUATION: Normal menstrual period = about 40 ml of blood.

- **AMENORRHEA:** No menstruation for 3 months or more.
  - **Primary Amenorrhea:** Failure of menarche
    - **Kallman's Syndrome:** Primary GnRH deficiency
    - **Turner's Syndrome:** XO
    - **Testicular Sensitization Syndrome:** Androgen insensitivity. Genotypic male may be diagnosed with testicular feminization when he presents as a teenager with primary amenorrhea.
    - Imperforate hymen
    - Congenital malformations of GU tract: Uterine agenesis, vaginal malformations.
  - **Secondary Amenorrhea:** Amenorrhea occurring any time after menarche has occurred.
    - Environmental Factors:

- Weight-reduction amenorrhea: Anorexia and related disorders, malnutrition.

- Psychogenic amenorrhea.

- Exercise-induced amenorrhea.

- Post-pill amenorrhea.

- Pituitary Disease:

  - **Prolactinoma**

  - **Sheehan Syndrome** = post-partum hemorrhage causing pituitary infarct from lack of blood-flow and increased pituitary demand.

- **Premature ovarian failure:** Menopause occurring before age 35. Can be caused oophoritis (mumps virus) or may be idiopathic.

- Polycystic Ovary Syndrome

- **Asherman's Syndrome:** Amenorrhea caused by intrauterine adhesions (synechiae) that obliterate part of the uterine cavity. This can occur subsequent to vigorous **dilatation and curettage (D&C)** of the endometrium.

- **HYPOMENORRHEA:** Decrease in volume of flow or duration of periods.

- **MENORRHAGIA, HYPERMENORRHEA:** Abnormally heavy volume of flow or abnormally long periods.

  o Most common causes: Uterine fibroids (leiomyomas), PIO, Endometriosis, IUD.

- **METRORRHAGIA:** Bleeding at mid-cycle. It is usually precipitated by the drop in estrogen that occurs after ovulation.

- **DYSMENORRHEA:** Painful menstruation. Symptoms = lower abdominal pain, nausea, vomiting, fatigue, diarrhea.

    o **Primary Dysmenorrhea:** Unexplained, idiopathic dysmenorrhea. Believed to be caused by high uterine levels of PGE2,
    o **Secondary Dysmenorrhea:** Endometriosis, PIO, imperforate hymen, uterine polyps, adhesions.
- **DYSFUNCTIONAL UTERINE BLEEDING (DUB):** Abnormal uterine bleeding in which no etiologic agent can be found after history and pelvic exam.

OTHER THINGS RELATING TO MENSTRUATION:

- **MENOPAUSE:**
- **PRE-MENSTRUAL SYNDROME:**

NON-MENSTRUAL VAGINAL BLEEDING: Bleeding not related to menstruation. When vaginal bleeding presents, we must determine whether it is menstrual or non-menstrual.

- **POST-MENOPAUSAL BLEEDING:** Consider **uterine cancer, cervical cancer.** Atrophic vaginitis if patient is not on ERT.

- **PREGNANCY:** Either intrauterine or ectopic, may cause bleeding for a variety of reasons.

- **BIRTH CONTROL METHODS:** IUD, **breakthrough bleeding** with pill.

PELVIC PAIN:

- **ACUTE PELVIC PAIN:**

    o **Mittelschmerz:** Pelvic pain occurring at mid-cycle and related to ovulation.

- o **Torsion of Ovary:** Cystic ovary can get large and twist on itself, cutting off its blood supply > acute-onset pelvic pain.

- o Ruptured tubal pregnancy.

- **CHRONIC PELVIC PAIN:**

  - o **Endometriosis:** Dysmenorrhea, dyspareunia, infertility. Often have chronic pelvic pain, associated with the location of the ectopic glandular tissue.

    - Pain of endometriosis tends to be constant, and tends to radiate to coccyx, lower back.
    - Onset of disease is usually between 25 and 40. Undifferentiated dysmenorrhea often presents younger than age 25.

URINARY TRACT INFECTIONS:

PREGNANCY and INFERTILITY:

- **EARLY PREGNANCY:** Common symptoms

  - o Secondary amenorrhea. Patient may also see reduced flow, or slight vaginal bleeding at time of normal period.
  - o Morning Sickness: Nausea and vomiting
  - o Breast tenderness
  - o Urinary frequency: cause may be anatomical or hormonal.
  - o Constipation
  - o Weight change: weight loss is common in early pregnancy, followed by weight gain later.

- **LATE PREGNANCY:**

  - o **Chloasma:** Characteristic darkening of skin around eyes, nose, cheeks. Darkening also occurs in areolae, skin between umbilicus and pubic ridge.

- o **Striae Gravidarum:** Stretch marks of pregnancy.

- o Spider angiomas may occur in skin, because of high estrogen.

- **PELVIC CHANGES WITH PREGNANCY:**

  - o **Chadwick's Sign:** Blue or purple discoloration of the vagina.

  - o **Leukorrhea:** Clear or white vaginal discharge with faint musty odour. It may occur during pregnancy or in other circumstances.

  - o **Goodell's Sign:** Bluish discoloration and softening of the cervix.

  - o **Braxton Hicks Contractions:** Painless uterine contractions occurring after the 28th week.

  - o **Quickening:** The first fetal movement of which the patient is aware. Normally occurs at 18 weeks during first pregnancy, and at 16 weeks in subsequent pregnancies.

- **HYDATIDIFORM MOLE:** Signs of a molar pregnancy:

  - o Uterus increases rapidly in size shortly after implantation.

  - o Persistent vaginal bleeding, no fetal movement, and no fetal heart tones by 12 weeks.

  - o Nausea and vomiting more intense than usual.

  - o Grape like clusters of tissues may be expelled through the vagina.

ABNORMALITIES in SEXUAL FUNCTION:

- **VAGINISMUS:** Spasmodic, guarding contraction of vagina upon attempt of intercourse. Often occurs subsequent to rape or trauma.

VAGINAL DISCHARGE and ITCHING:

- **PHYSIOLOGIC DISCHARGE:** Clear or white discharge occurring at midcycle.

- **TRICHOMONAS VAGINA/IS:**

    - Discharge: Gray, foamy discharge having bad odour.
    - Mucosa: Red, strawberry cervix.
    - Confirm: Confirm with **wet mount** (saline suspension microscopy).

- **GONORRHEA:**

    - Discharge: Profuse mucoid discharge with foul odour.
    - Mucosa: Red, tender mucosa.
    - Confirm: Confirm with culture.

- **GARDNERELLA VAGINA/IS:** Also called **Non-specific vaginitis.** Co-infection with anaerobes usually also occurs.

    - Discharge: Gray or white, fishy odor
    - Mucosa: Normal
    - Confirm: **Clue cells** = large epithelial cells with many coccobacilli adherent to them.

- **CHLAMYDIA:**

    - Discharge: Little, yellow, mucous and pus in cervical canal.
    - Mucosa: Cervical erosion.
    - Confirm: FA stain of smear shows **elementary bodies.**

- **CANDIDA ALBICANS:** Yeast infection.

    - Discharge: White, cottage-cheese like.
    - Mucosa: White patches stuck to a red base.

- o   Confirm: KOH preparation, look for pseudohypha.

- **ATROPHIC VAGINITIS:** Estrogen deficiency

- o   Discharge: Little discharge, some blood.

- o   Mucosa: Atrophic, pale or red.

- o   Confirm: history, age.

***PELVIC RELAXATION*:** Loss of pelvis support due to atrophy of muscular viscera.

- **URETHROCELE:** Urethra herniates into the vaginal canal.

- **CYSTOCELE:** Bladder herniates into the vaginal canal.

- **RECTOCELE:** Rectum herniates into the vaginal canal.

- **UTERINE PROLAPSE:** Descent of the uterus into the vaginal canal. Graded from 1 (mild) to 3 (uterus descends past the vulva).

HIRSUTISM

PHYSICAL EXAM

7.0 MUSCULOSKELETAL

EPIDEMIOLOGY:

- **COMMON MUSCULOSKELETAL DISEASES BY AGE:**
  - Childhood: Juvenile RA, Rheumatic Fever
  - Young adult: Reiter's Syndrome, SLE
  - Middle Age: Fibrositis
  - Old Age: Osteoarthritis

- **COMMON MUSCULOSKELETAL DISEASES BY SEX:**
  - Male: Gout
  - Female: SLE, RA

- **COMMON MUSCULOSKELETAL DISEASES BY RACE:**
  - Black: Sarcoidosis, SLE
  - White: Polymyalgia Rheumatica

SYMPTOMS:

REITER'S SYNDROME:

- Symptoms: **Conjunctivitis, Urethritis, Arthritis.**
- Signs:
  - **Keratoderma Blennorrhagia:** Rash on palms and soles.
  - **Circinate Balanitis:** Circular rash on penis.
  - **Sausage fingers:** Swelling of the tendon sheath of the hands.

PSORIATIC ARTHRITIS: Arthritis occurring with Psoriasis.

- Signs:
    - **Sausage fingers**: Swelling of the tendon sheath of the hands.
    - DIP joints may be inflamed unilaterally.

GOUT:

- Symptoms:
    - **Podagra:** Severe gouty pain at the base of the great toe.

RHEUMATIC FEVER:

- Symptoms:
    - **Migratory Pain:** Typical finding. Pain moving from joint to joint.
- **Jones Criteria:** Diagnostic criteria for Rheumatic Fever. Two major criteria, or one major and two minor criteria are required.
    - **Major Criteria:**
        - **Carditis:** Myocarditis, Pericarditis
        - Polyarthritis
        - **Chorea:** Purposeless movements of various muscle groups
        - **Erythema Marginatum**: Pink, circular rash on trunk on proximal arms.
        - **Subcutaneous Nodules:** Granulomatous nodules on extensor surfaces, often associated with cardiac involvement.
    - **Minor Criteria:**
        - History, Symptoms:

- History of previous rheumatic fever or rheumatic heart disease.
- Arthralgia
- Fever

• Labs:

• Acute phase reactants: increased ESR, C-Reactive Protein, leukocytosis.

• ECG abnormalities

• Recent streptococcal infection.

GONORRHEA, DISSEMINATED (Gonococcal Arthritis):

- Symptoms:
  - **Migratory Pain:** Typical finding. Pain moving from joint to joint.

RHEUMATOID ARTHRITIS:

- Symptoms:
  - **Morning stiffness:** Pain in the morning, which tends to loosen up as the day progresses.
  - **Fatigue:** During the day, fatigue sets in. The earlier the fatigue sets in, the worse is the RA.
- Signs: The proximal (PIP and MCP) joints are characteristically more involved than the DIP joints.
  - Synovial Thickening – swelling of joints.
  - Entire phalanx may deviate laterally or medially.

- o **Boutonniere Deformity, Swan-Neck Deformity, Ulnar Deviation:** Characteristic deformities of hands and wrists seen in Rheumatoid Arthritis.

OSTEOARTHRITIS: Degenerative arthritis.

- Symptoms:
  - o Pain usually gets worse as the day progresses, leading to fatigue in the afternoon.
- Signs: The distal (DIP) joints are characteristically more involved than the PIP joints.
  - o Distal phalanx may deviate laterally.
  - o **Heberden's Nodes:** Bony overgrowths on the dorsum of the DIP joints, typical of osteoarthritis.

SYSTEMIC LUPUS ERYTHEMATOSUS (SLE): Diagnostic Criteria. 4 of 11 at any time is diagnostic.

- **MALAR RASH**
- **DISCOID RASH**
- **PHOTOSENSITIVITY**
- **ORAL ULCERS**
- **ARTHRITIS**
- **SEROSITIS (PLEURITIS, PERICARDITIS)**
- **RENAL DISORDER**
- **NEUROLOGIC DISORDER (SEIZURES, PSYCHOSIS)**
- **HEMATOLOGIC** (anemia, leukopenia, lymphopenia, thrombocytopenia).
- **IMMUNOLOGIC** (elevated anti-DNA, LE-Prep, or biological false positive for Syphilis (RPR))
- **ANTINUCLEAR ANTIBODY (ANA)**

SYMPTOMS:

PAIN:

- Generally, the deeper the musculoskeletal structure, the more diffuse the pain.
    - Pain from bone is deep or boring pain.
    - Pain from periosteum is more localized.
- **REFERRED PAIN:** Don't forget the Ddx of CAD in shoulder pain.
- **ARTHRALGIA:** Defined as joint pains without objective signs of inflammation. It is caused by many processes, both inflammatory and non-inflammatory.
- **ARTHRITIS:** Joint inflammation.

STIFFNESS:

WEAKNESS:

- **WEAKNESS:** Loss of strength, due to mechanical or neurological impairment.
- **FATIGUE:** Poor endurance.

INSPECTION:

PALPATION: May find the following abnormalities on palpation:

Swelling

- Synovial thickening (pannus formation) is characteristic of RA.

- Swelling of tendon-sheath (sausage-shaped digit) occurs in Reiter's Syndrome and Psoriatic Arthritis.

- **Effusions:** Fluid is most commonly found in the knee

DEFORMITY

- **GANGLIA:** Fluid-filled cysts found along joint capsules, usually in the wrist.
- **RHEUMATOID NODULES:** Firm nodules found on extensor surfaces of bony prominences. They contain mononuclear cells and fibrosis.
- **GOUTY TOPHI:** Joint nodules associated with urate deposits.
- **BURSITIS:** Inflammation of the bursa in the knee or elbow.

ERYTHEMA AND WARMTH: Especially in inflammatory or infectious processes.

LIMITATION OF RANGE OF MOTION:

TENDERNESS: The subjective sensation of pain upon pressure.

- Grading:
    - 0: No tenderness
    - 1: Patient says it is tender
    - 2: Patient says it is tender and winces
    - 3: Patient says it is tender, winces, and pulls back
    - 4: Patient will not allow palpations
- Joint noises or locking

AUSCULTATION:

- **CREPITUS:** Grating or grinding sensation felt by patient or heard by examiner. Rubbing of bones due to degeneration of articular cartilage.

- **CRACKING, SNAPPING:** Snapping of joints is usually not pathologic, unless it occurs repeatedly.

- **CLICKING:** May indicate an abnormality when it occurs in TMJ joint.

MUSCLE STRENGTH: **Graded on a scale from 5 to 0**

- **5:** Full strength

- **4:** Strength against gravity and added resistance.

- **3:** Strength only against gravity, not added resistance.

- **2:** Muscle contraction occurs, but not sufficient to overcome gravity.

- **1:** Muscle contracts with little or no movement.

- **0:** No muscle contraction.

RANGE OF MOTION

- **ACTIVE RANGE OF MOTION:** Voluntary movement.

- **PASSIVE RANGE OF MOTION:** Examiner moves the joint.

- **GONIOMETER:** Device used to measure angles, to assess the range of motion of a joint.

- **UNSTABLE JOINT:** Excessive joint motion (excessive extension) of the knee may be seen in osteoarthritis.

HEAD EXAM:

- TMJ Abnormalities are caused by dental malocclusion, trauma to the jaw, RA.

NECK (CERVICAL SPINE):

- Arthritis may limit rotation or lateral flexion of the neck.

SHOULDER:

- **ROTATOR CUFF INJURY:** Pain or spasm in mid-abduction is a sign of rotator cuff injury. This is due to degeneration in the subacromial bursa, resulting in friction between the supraspinatus muscle and acromial process at mid-abduction.
    - Arm can't rise above about 90, the extent to which the Deltoid can abduct it.

- **ADHESIVE CAPSULITIS (FROZEN SHOULDER):** Unilateral diffuse, dull, aching pain.
    - Tenderness is diffuse.

- **AC DEGENERATIVE ARTHRITIS:** Maybe from trauma. It hurts upon movement of scapula.

- **BICIPITAL TENDINITIS (IMPINGEMENT SYNDROME):** Inflammation of the tendon of the supraspinatus muscle.

- **CALCIFIC TENDINITIS:** Prolonged inflammation of the supraspinatus tendon, with resulting calcification.

ELBOW:

- **TENNIS ELBOW:** Tender and inflamed **lateral epicondyle,** resulting from repeated extension. Patient will experience pain when asked to extend the elbow against resistance.

- **GOLFER'S ELBOW:** Inflammation of the **medial epicondyle.** Typically shows pain when asked to lift with the palms facing upward (volar aspect).

WRIST:

- Diseases:
    - **DEQUERVAIN'S TENOSYNOVITIS:** Involves the extensor tendon of the thumb. Ask patient to apply pressure with thumb against the forefinger, and pain will result.
    - **GANGLION:** Cyst caused by herniated synovium into soft tissues.
    - **CARPAL TUNNEL SYNDROME:** Compression of median nerve through carpal tunnel.

        - **Phalen's Test:** Ask patient to flex each wrist at 90 for one minute. Positive test occurs if numbness and tingling over median distribution results.

        - **Tinel's Sign:** Tingling shots of pain over median nerve upon percussion of the wrist.

    - **DUPUYTREN'S CONTRACTURE:** Fibrous contraction of the palmar aponeurosis.

        - May be found in RA, alcoholism, or familial.

- Signs:

    - **Bouchard's Nodes:** Swelling of the PIP joints, which is less common than swelling of the DIP joints.
    - **Heberden's Nodes:** Bony overgrowths on the dorsum of the DIP joints, typical of osteoarthritis.
    - **Boutonniere Deformity:** Flexion contracture of the PIP joint, with hyperextension of the DIP joint. Caused by injury or RA.
    - **Swan Neck Deformity:** Hyperextended PIP joints and flexed DIP joints. May accompany RA.

SPINE:

- **SCOLIOSIS:** Lateral curvature of spine. When bending over, muscular prominences on one side of the back is more prominent than the other side.

- **STRAIGHT BACK SYNDROME:** Lack of normal thoracic kyphosis.

- **DOWAGER'S HUMP:** Marked kyphosis of dorsal spine in elderly women.

- **ANKYLOSING SPONDYLITIS:** RA-like disease affecting the lower spine and sacroiliac joints.

- **LUMBOSACRAL STRAIN:** Lower back pain from obesity and or poor posture.

- **HERNIATED NUCLEUS PULPOSUS:**

- **SCIATICA:**

HIP:

- If one leg is shorter than the other as measured from ASIS to ankle, hip disease is likely.

- **TRENDELENBURG TEST:** Have patient stand on one foot. The contralateral hip should pull upward. If it doesn't, and the same hip on which patient is standing instead pulls downward, then that is a positive test and is indicative of hip disease.

- **ANTALGIC GAIT:** Walking funny (limping) in order to avoid pain in the hip.

KNEE:

- **BAKER'S CYST:** Extension of the synovium into the popliteal space. Felt on posterior knee.

- **OSGOOD-SCHLATTER DISEASE:** Partial separation of the quadriceps femoris tendon at the tibial tuberosity, making the tibial tuberosity swollen and tender. Seen in adolescents.

- **GENU VALGUS:** Knock-kneed. Knees bend inward.

- **GENU VARUS:** Bowlegged. Knees bend outward.

- **GENU RECURVATUM:** Excessive extension of the knee.

ANKLE and FEET:

- **BUNION:** Swelling of the great toe. Usually, valgus is seen too.

- **FLAT FOOT (PES P/ANUS):** Relaxation of longitudinal arches, resulting in flattening of the arch of the foot. Patients tend to wear down the soles of their shoes on the medial side.

- **HIGH ARCHES (PES CAVUS):** Have excessive wear on their soles at the base of the heel and under the metatarsal heads.

- **HEEL SPUR:** Tenderness may happen at the insertion of the plantar longitudinal tendon on the calcaneus.

- **MORTON NEUROMA:** Pinching of fibrous neuromas between metatarsal heads, resulting severe burning pain.

8.0 NEUROLOGICAL

NEUROLOGIC SYMPTOMS:

HEADACHE:

- **MIGRAINE HEADACHE:** Often preceded by aura, and associated with weakness, numbness, and paresthesia.

- **TENSION HEADACHE:** Usually is frontal or occipital. Tends to be recurrent.

- **CLUSTER HEADACHE:** In males, occurring at night, 2-3 hours after falling asleep. Symptoms are intense unilateral orbital pain (over one eye), with lacrimation, rhinorrhea, flushing. Usually lasts about 1 hour.

- **CAUSES of SECONDARY HEADACHE:**

    o **Meningismus:** Stiff neck. If it occurs with the "worst headache of my life", then you should be suspicious of **subarachnoid hemorrhage.**

    o **Projectile Vomiting:** Headache with projectile vomiting, occurring in morning, usually means increased intracranial pressure.

    o **Transient loss of Consciousness:** Headache accompanied by transient loss of consciousness should raise question of **stroke.**

SYNCOPE and LOSS of CONSCIOUSNESS:

SEIZURES:

- Types of Seizures:

    o **Complex Partial Seizures:** Patients commonly have feelings of fear or Déjà vu associated with complex partial seizures.

- o **Grand Mal Seizures:** Tonic-clonic, often with loss of autonomic control.

- o **Petit Mal Seizures:** Lasting for a short period of time – only a few seconds.

- **CAUSES of SEIZURE:**

  - o Adolescents (12-20): Idiopathic **(Epilepsy),** Trauma, Drug and alcohol withdrawal.
  - o Young Adults (20-35): Trauma, alcoholism, brain tumour
  - o Older adults (35+): **brain tumour**, CVA, metabolic disorders, electrolyte imbalances (**hyponatremia,** hypoglycemia, uremia).

- **CHANGES in VISION:**

  - o **Amaurosis Fugax**: Transient, painless loss of vision in one eye, due to ischemic changes in retina. Usually due to **carotid artery stenosis** or some form of retinal artery occlusion.

    - Other symptoms, such as weakness, paresthesia, often accompany the Amaurosis Fugax.

  - o **Retrobulbar Neuritis:** Occurs in **Multiple Sclerosis** and may cause transient loss of vision in one eye.

- **CHANGES in HEARING:**

- **CHANGES in SPEECH:**

  - o **Dysarthria:** Difficulty in articulating words.

  - o **Dysphonia:** Difficulty speaking due to impaired phonation ability.

  - o **Aphasia:** Inability to produce (**motor aphasia**) or understand (**receptive aphasia**) meaningful speech.

- **PARALYSIS or WEAKNESS: Paresis** is intermittent weakness.

    o   CAUSES of Paresis:

    - Myasthenia Gravis (fatigable weakness).

    - **Hypokalemia** can result in periodic paralysis.

    - **Transient ischemic attacks (TIA's):** Recurrent Transient weaknesses in an upper extremity, accompanied by numbness and paresthesia.

    - Peripheral neuropathies.

    - Polymyositis or dermatomyositis.

- **NUMBNESS and PARESTHESIA:**

    o   Hypocalcemia, hypomagnesemia.

    o   Hyperventilation syndrome.

    o   Paraneoplastic syndrome.

    o   Medications: isoniazid, metronidazole.

- **CHANGES in MOOD and SLEEP PATTERN:**

- **ALCOHOL and DRUG USE, SEXUAL HISTORY:**

    o   Sexual history: In the neuro exam, may inquire about it to evaluate risk of HIV encephalopathy.

    o   Alcoholism manifests a lot of neurological symptoms (Wernicke, beriberi, peripheral neuropathies).

NEUROLOGIC EXAM:

ASSESSMENT of MOTOR FUNCTION: Sometimes pluses and minuses can be used for even finer grading.

- **0:** No contraction; paralysis.
- **1:** Trace of contraction.
- **2:** Moves if gravity is eliminated.
- **3:** Moves against gravity.
- **4:** Moves against gravity and against some resistance.
- **5:** Normal strength.

MOTOR ABNORMALITIES:

- **HYSTERIA:** To test whether weakness in the leg is from hysteria or is organic, put a hand on both limbs and have the patient lift one limb against the hand's resistance.
    - If the cause of motor weakness is organic, then examiner should feel the other leg move in the opposite direction in compensation.
    - If it is hysteria, then the other leg remains still.

- **FASCICULATIONS:** Twitching in resting muscles. May be normal if they are occasional or precipitated by cold. They may be a sign of **Amyotrophic Lateral Sclerosis (ALS)** if they are accompanied by weakness.

- **TICS:** Normal movements of muscle groups (such as winking or grinning) occurring involuntarily, as in Tourette's Syndrome.

- **TETANY:** Involuntary muscle spasms.
    - Causes: Tetanus, hypocalcemia, hypomagnesemia, hyperventilation syndrome.

- o **Chvostek's Sign:** Tap over facial nerve anterior to ear, and look for contraction of the facial muscles, especially shutting of eyes.

- o **Trousseau's Phenomenon**: Inflate a blood-pressure cuff to systolic pressure and maintain for 1-2 minutes. Induction of carpal-pedal spasm indicates latent tetany.

- **TREMORS:** Oscillating movements caused by involuntary contractions of muscle groups.

SENSORY EVALUATION

- **PERIPHERAL NEUROPATHIES:** tend to occur in hand-and-glove distribution – at the distal ends of the extremities.

- **PAIN:** Upon pinprick, patient may experience **hypalgesia** (reduced pain), hyperalgesia, or analgesia (no pain).

- **LIGHT TOUCH:**

  - o Hypesthesia = Impaired light touch sensation. Also related to light-touch are hyperesthesia, paresthesia, and anesthesia (no light touch).

- **SENSORY EXTINCTION:** In parietal lobe lesions, if you put a pinprick on both sides of the body of a patient simultaneously, the patient will not perceive the prick on the affected side of the lesion. If the pins are placed sequentially, then the patient still retains normal sensation on both sides.

STEREOGNOSIS: Being able to identify objects with your eyes closed.

CEREBELLAR FUNCTION:

- **DYSERGIA:** Improper coordinated function of a muscle group.

- **DYSMETRIA:** Inability to properly gauge the distance between two points. Tested with finger-to-nose movements.
- **DYSDIADOCHOKINESIA:** Inability to do rapid alternating movements.
- **SCANNING SPEECH:** Prolonged separation of syllables, often seen with cerebellar dysfunction.
- **GAIT DISTURBANCES:**
    - Cerebellar Lesions: Central cerebellar lesion shows unsteady gait, but conventional cerebellar signs may be normal.
    - **Posterior Columns Lesions:** Loss of proprioception results in unsteady gait when eyes are closed, but relatively normal gait when eyes are open.
    - **Festinating Gait:** Parkinsonian gait, shuffling walk.
- **ROMBERG TEST:** Patient can't maintain balance with legs tight together, with eyes closed.
- **TITUBATION:** Body tremor when standing or walking, sign of cerebellar disease.

REFLEXES:

DEEP TENDON REFLEXES:

- **UPPER EXTREMITY:**
    - **Biceps Reflex:** Elbow flexion.
    - **Triceps Reflex:** Forearm extension.
    - **Brachioradialis** Reflex: Tap distal radius > flexion and partial supination of the forearm.

- **LOWER EXTREMITY:**
    - **Patellar Reflex:** Contraction of Quadriceps (strongest muscles in body) and extension of leg.
    - **Suprapatellar Reflex:** Above the knee; same response.
    - **Achilles Reflex:** Causes plantarflexion of foot.

- **REFLEX GRADING:**
  - 0: Complete absence
  - 1: Diminished
  - 2: **Normal Reflex**
  - 3: Hyperactive reflex
  - 4: Clonus

- **SUPERFICIAL REFLEXES:**
  - Upper Abdominal: Ipsilateral contraction of abdominal muscles on the stroked side.
  - Lower Abdominal: Ipsilateral contraction of abdominal muscles on the stroked side.
  - Cremasteric: Stroke inner thigh ------> elevation of testes.

- **BRAINSTEM REFLEXES:**
  - Corneal Reflex
  - Pupillary Light Reflex
  - Gag Reflex

- **ABNORMAL REFLEXES:**
  - **Babinski Sign:** Stroke bottom of the foot------> fanning (eversion) of big toe.
  - **Chaddock's Reflex:** When the external malleolar skin area is irritated, extension of the great toe occurs in cases of organic disease of the corticospinal reflex paths.
  - **Oppenheim's Sign:** Scratch inner side of leg > extension of toes. Sign of cerebral irritation.

- o **Gordon's Sign:** Squeeze the calf muscles and note the response of the great toe. Fanning or extension is considered abnormal.

- o **Hoffman's Sign:** Flexion of the terminal phalanx of the thumb and of the second and third phalanges of one or more of the fingers when the volar surface of the terminal phalanx of the fingers is flicked.

  - It is significant for pyramidal tract disease when it is unilateral. If it is bilateral than the meaning is uncertain.

ABSENCE OF SUPERFICIAL REFLEXES: Unilateral suppression of superficial reflexes often results from upper motor lesions subsequent to a CVA.

PRIMITIVE REFLEXES: Presence of primitive reflexes is often a sign of **frontal lobe** lesions.

- **SUCK REFLEX:** Gently tap or rub the upper lift ------> elicit a reflexive sucking or puckering response.
- **GRASP REFLEX:** Stroke the patient's palm, causing him to grasp your fingers. A positive test occurs when the patient does not let go of your fingers.
- **PALMOMENTAL SIGN:** Rub the thenar eminence   > elicit reflexive contraction of the muscles of the chin.

CRANIAL NERVE EVALUATION:

CN I: OLFACTORY

- TEST: Have patient identify objects by smell.

- **ABNORMAL:**

  - o Head trauma with fracture of cribriform plate

  - o Neoplasm in anterior fossa: meningioma

CN II: OPTIC

- **TEST:** Visual acuity, funduscopic exam
- **ABNORMAL:** Lots of causes of blindness

CN III: OCULOMOTOR

- **TEST:**
  - Have patient move eyes through all fields of vision. Intact 3rd nerve means that eyes can move medially, superiorly, and inferiorly.
  - **Pupillary Reflex:** Check for pupillary response to light in same eye and contralateral eye.
  - **Ptosis:** Ptosis may occur due to 3rd nerve palsy.
- **ABNORMAL:**
  - Unilateral CN-III Palsy: Subarachnoid hemorrhage resulting from aneurysm, diabetes, atherosclerosis.
  - Homer's Syndrome: Usually occurs from **bronchogenic carcinoma (Pancoast Tumor)** impinging on the Superior Cervical Ganglion.

CN IV: TROCHLEAR

- **TEST:**
- **ABNORMAL:**

CN V: TRIGEMINAL

- **TEST:**
  - Sensory: Check corneal reflex. Test facial sensation with eyes closed.
  - Motor: Have patient clench teeth and palpate masseter muscle.

- **ABNORMAL:**

  - Lost Corneal Reflex: Tumour of the cerebellopontine angle.

  - **Tic Douloureux**: Irritative lesions of the CN V sensory roots.

  - Spasm of muscles of mastication: tetanus, adverse reaction to Phenothiazines.

CN VI: ABDUCENS

- **TEST:** Look laterally.

- **ABNORMAL:**

  - Diabetes, atherosclerosis, increased ICP, neoplasm.

CN VII: FACIAL

- **TEST:** Have patient smile, blink, frown, wrinkle forehead.

- **ABNORMAL: Bell's Palsy**

  - **Central Lesion of VII:** The supratrochlear muscles are spared, as they receive bilateral innervation from both facial nerves. Below the eyes, the contralateral side will be paralyzed.

  - **Peripheral Lesion of VII:** There is an entire facial hemiplegia, with the paralysis occurring on the contralateral side.

CN VIII: VESTIBULOCOCHLEAR

- **TEST:** Standard hearing and vestibular tests.

- **ABNORMAL:** A variety of disorders

CNIX: GLOSSOPHARYNGEAL

- **TEST:** Have patient open mouth and say "Aaahhh".

- **ABNORMAL:** See Vagus N. below.

CN X: VAGUS

- **TEST:** Have patient open mouth and say "Aaahhh".

- **ABNORMAL:**

    o Aortic Aneurysm, Bronchogenic Carcinoma may damage the recurrent laryngeal nerve.

    o Uvula will deviate toward the damaged side.

CN XI: SPINAL ACCESSORY

- **TEST:** Have patient shrug shoulders.

- **ABNORMAL:** Polymyositis

CN XII: HYPOGLOSSAL

- **TEST:** Have patient stick out tongue.

PHYSICAL SIGNS

Sign	Description, Finding	Indication
Doll's Eye Sign	Dissociation between movement of the eyes and of the head. Eyes moves up and head moves down.	
Babinski's Sign	Fanning of big toe when you stroke the plantar aspect of the foot.	CNS: Pyramidal Tract Lesion
Chaddock's Sign	Great toe fanning when you touch the external malleolar skin.	CNS: Corticospinal tract lesions
Eyelash Sign	Stroking eyelash produces no movement of lids.	CNS: Organic stroke.
	Stroking eyelash produces movement of lids.	CNS: Functional hysteria
Hoffman's Sign	Nipping nail of middle finger cause flexion of terminal phalanx of thumb. Unilaterally.	CNS: Pyramidal Tract Disease
Clenched Fist (Levine's) Sign	Holding clenched fist over chest to describe constricting, pressing pain.	CV: Angina Pectoris
de Musset's Sign	Rhythmic jerking movement of the head.	CV: Aortic Insufficiency
Ewart's Sign	Dullness, bronchial breathing, bronchophony over the angle of the left scapula.	CV: Pericardial effusion
Hamman's Sign	Crunching sound synchronous with heartbeat.	CV: Mediastinal Emphysema, Pneumopericardium
Hill's Sign	Exaggerated femoral artery systolic pressure (60 to 100 mm Hg higher) over brachial systolic pressure.	CV: Aortic Insufficiency
Homan's Sign	Pain in back of calf or knee when foot is dorsiflexed.	CV: Thrombosis in veins of calf

Sign	Description, Finding	Indication
Kussmaul's Sign	Paradoxical increase in jugular venous distension when patient inspires.	CV: Cardiac Tamponade
Osier's Sign	Painful erythematous swellings in skin and subcutaneous tissues of hands and feet.	CV: Endocarditis
Joffroy's Sign	No forehead wrinkling when the eyeballs are rolled upward.	Endocrine: Grave's Disease
Mobius Sign	Impaired ocular convergence (accommodation)	Endocrine: Grave's Disease
Stellwag's Sign	Infrequent and incomplete blinking.	Endocrine: Grave's Disease
Kestenbaum's Sign	Decrease in number of arterioles crossing optic disk margins.	Eye: Optic Atrophy
Marcus Gunn Pupillary Sign	Flashlight swung from one eye to the other eye, then both pupils dilate (when nerve defects they should constrict).	Eye: Cataract, optic nerve defects
Cullen's Sign	Periumbilical darkening of the skin	GI: Intraperitoneal haemorrhage, from haemorrhagic pancreatitis
Grey Turner's Sign	Local discoloration of the skin of the loins.	GI: Acute haemorrhagic pancreatitis
Groove Sign	Firm nodes in groin above and below inguinal ligament, with a groove along the ligament.	GI: Lymphogranuloma Venereum
Kehr's Sign	Violent pain in the left shoulder	GI: Ruptured Spleen
Puddle Sign	Patient gets on all fours, and palpating at one end allows auscultation at the other end of the abdomen. Stethoscope moves from most dependent position gradually contralaterally.	GI: Ascites

Sign	Description, Finding	Indication
Rovsing's Sign	Pain in right abdomen at McBurney's Point when pressure is exerted on left abdomen.	GI: Appendicitis
Barany's Sign	Irrigate ear with cold water: should lead to nystagmus on opposite side. Irrigate ear with warm water: should lead to nystagmus on same side. This sign shows no nystagmus.	Head and Neck: Labyrinthine disease, such as Meniere's Disease
Battle's Sign	Postauricular ecchymosis.	Head and Neck: fracture of the base of the of the skull.
Brudzinski's Sign	(1) Contralateral leg reflex: passive flexion of leg on one side elicits reflex on the opposite side. (2) Passively flex neck, and hips and knees flex spontaneously.	Infectious: Meningitis
Kernig's Sign	Patient lies on back and flexes thigh upward, then complete extension of leg is impossible.	Infectious: Meningitis
Pastia's Sign	Haemorrhagic transverse lines at bend of elbow, wrist, or Inguinal region. It persists after desquamation.	Infectious: Scarlet Fever
Romberg's Sign	Close eyes and lose gait; ataxia.	Infectious: Tabes Dorsalis
Winterbottom's Sign	Swelling of posterior cervical lymph nodes.	Infectious: African Sleeping Sickness (Trypanosomiasis)
Chvostek's Sign	Facial irritability. Unilateral spasm induced by tap over the facial nerve.	Muscular: Tetany
Trousseau's Sign	Upper arm compressed by a tourniquet or blood-pressure cuff causes carpal spasm.	Muscular: Tetany
Braxton Hicks Contractions	Irregular uterine contractions after third month of pregnancy.	OB/GYN: Pregnancy

Sign	Description, Finding	Indication
Chadwick's Sign	Bluish discoloration of cervix and vagina.	OB/GYN: Pregnancy
Drawer Sign	Forward sliding (anterior cruciate) or backward sliding (posterior cruciate) of the tibia.	Skeletal: Disruption of anterior (forward slide) or posterior (backward slide) cruciate ligaments of knee.
Lasegue's Sign	When patient is supine with hip flexed up, dorsiflexion of the ankle causes pain.	Skeletal: Sciatic Nerve irritation (Sciatica)
Nikolsky's Sign	Sliding pressure of thumb pressed against skin separates outer layer from basal dermis.	Skin: Pemphis Vulgaris

TABLE OF PHYSICAL FINDINGS

Finding	Description, Comments	Associated Disease(s)
Adie's Pupil	Similar to Argyll Robertson Pupil, except that accommodation is also impaired. May also see impaired deep tendon reflexes.	Adie's Syndrome
Angioid Streaks	FUNDUSCOPIC: Pigmented lines radiating outward from the optic disc.	Pseudoxanthoma Elasticum
Angiokeratomas	Purplish; red papules, on lower abdomen, groin, or scrotum.	Fabry's Disease: Hereditary Glycolipid Lipidosis.
Arcus Senilis	Grey band of opacity around the cornea, a normal finding with aging.	
Argyll Robertson Pupils	No pupillary light reflex, but accommodation is intact.	Neurosyphilis
Argyll Robertson Pupil	(1) Weak or absent direct pupillary reflex, (2) Retained ability to accommodate for near vision, (3) Failed pupillary dilation after atropine administration.	Tabes Dorsalis (Neurosyphilis)
Arteriovenous (AV) Nicking	FUNDUSCOPIC: Arteriolar narrowing and compression of veins, where the arteries cross the veins. Due to sclerotic changes in both arteries and veins.	Hypertensive Retinopathy: Stage II
Babinski's Sign	Fanning of big toe when you stroke the plantar aspect of the foot.	Pyramidal Tract Lesion
Blue coloured Sclerae	Thin collagen in sclera makes venous blood visible.	Osteogenesis Imperfecta
Borborygmi	Loud, high-pitched bowel sounds, often associated with rushes.	Small Bowel Obstruction
Boutonniere Deformity	Flexion contracture of PIP joints, plus hyperextension of DIP joint, as if one were pushing a button through a button hole.	Rheumatoid Arthritis

Finding	Description, Comments	Associated Disease(s)
Braxton Hicks Contractions	Painless uterine contractions occurring after the 28th week.	Pregnancy
Brown coloured Sclera	May also be seen in normal black men.	Alkaptonuria
Brushfield_Spots	Grey white spots on iris.	Down's Syndrome
Buffalo Hump	Fatty deposit over C7	Cushing's Syndrome
Bullous Myringitis	Bullous inflammation of the tympanic membrane, visible through the otoscope.	Mycoplasma Pneumonia
Cafe Au Lait Spots	Neurofibromatosis	Von Recklinghausen Disease: Neurofibromatosis Type I
Chaddock's Reflex	When the external malleolar skin area is irritated, extension of the great toe occurs.	Pyramidal Tract Lesion
Chadwick's Sign	Bluish or purple discolour of the vagina.	Pregnancy
Cherry-Red Spot of Macula	FUNDUSCOPIC: Abnormally dim retinal background, with redness on macula.	Tay-Sach's Disease, Retina Artery Occlusion
Cheyne-Stokes Respiration	Cyclic alternations between apnoea and hyperpnea, in which PC02 fluctuates and is unstable. It occurs when the respiratory centres of the brain become insensitive to changes in CO2.	Congestive Heart Failure (CHF) Also Uraemia, Meningitis, Pneumonia
Chvostek's Sign	Tap over facial nerve anterior to ear, and look for contraction of the facial muscles, especially shutting of eyes.	Tetany
Circinate Balanus	Circular rash around penis.	Reiter's Syndrome
Clubbing	Characteristic down turning of fingernails.	Central Cyanosis from any cause, Infective Endocarditis

Finding	Description, Comments	Associated Disease(s)
Copper wiring	FUNDUSCOPIC: Blood may appear orange rather than red, due to arteriolar narrowing.	Hypertensive Retinopathy
Corneal Arcus (Arcus Senilis)	Opaque greyish ring around cornea resulting from fatty deposits.	Atherosclerosis in young people; may be normal finding in old people.
Corrigan's Pulse	Collapsing Pulse, or a brisk pule with large volume.	Aortic Insufficiency
Cotton Wool Exudates	FUNDUSCOPIC: soft exudates caused by ischemia to nerve-fibre layers.	Hypertensive Retinopathy: Stage III
Dot Haemorrhage	FUNDUSCOPIC: haemorrhage appearance characteristic of diabetes.	Diabetic Retinopathy
Dowager's Hump	Kyphosis of thoracic spine, from vertebral micro-fractures.	Osteoporosis
Duroziez Murmur	Bruit heard over the femoral artery, during both systole and diastole. Should be heard coincident with Corrigan's Pulse.	Aortic Insufficiency
Erythema Marginatum	Large erythematous patches with jagged edges and central clearing. One of the Major Jones Criteria.	Rheumatic Fever
Exophthalmos	Bulging eyes.	Grave's Disease. Also – Acromegaly, Cavernous Sinus Thrombosis.
Fasciculations	Muscle twitching due to spontaneous repetitive firing of motor nerves. It can occur normally in the cold.	Amyotrophic Lateral Sclerosis (ALS), or other upper motor demyelinating diseases
Flail Chest	One side of the chest moves paradoxically relative to the other side. Caused by multiple Rib fractures.	Injury: Rib fractures
Flame-shaped haemorrhages	FUNDUSCOPIC: Haemorrhage appearance characteristic of hypertension.	Hypertensive Retinopathy

Finding	Description, Comments	Associated Disease(s)
Gibbus Deformity	Sharp change of angle of spine, instead of gradual change of angle.	Pott's Disease: Tuberculous Spondylitis
Goodell's Sign	Bluish discoloration plus softening of the cervix.	Pregnancy
Grasp Reflex	Stroke the patient's palm, causing him to grasp your fingers. A positive test occurs when the patient does not let go of your fingers.	Frontal Lobe Lesion: A primitive reflex.
Grey Turner's Sign	Ecchymoses on the abdomen.	Fulminant Acute Pancreatitis, carrying a grave prognosis.
Hamman's Sign	Crunching, crackling sound over chest heard synchronous with the heartbeat.	Mediastinal Emphysema: Air in mediastinum, after thoracic surgery or trauma. Rare cause: Oesophageal rupture (Boerhaave's Syndrome)
Heberden's Nodes	Bone spurs appearing over DIP joints, on the dorsum of the finger.	Osteoarthritis
Hoffman's Sign	Nipping nail of middle finger causes flexion of terminal phalanx of thumb, unilaterally.	Pyramidal Tract Lesion
Hoffman's Sign	Flick the terminal phalanx of a finger------> flexion of the terminal phalanges of thumb, first, and/or second fingers.	Pyramidal Tract Disease: Only when the finding is unilateral. If the finding is bilateral then the meaning is uncertain.
Hutchinson's Triad	Classical triad of Interstitial Keratitis, Deafness, Notched Teeth	Congenital Syphilis in the new-born
Impaired Convergence	Inability to normally focus and look inward for extreme near vision	Grave's Disease

Finding	Description, Comments	Associated Disease(s)
Janeway Lesions	Non-tender, raised erythematous nodules on the palms.	Vasculitis
Keratoderma Blennorrhagia	Rash on the palms and soles.	Reiter's Syndrome
Koplik's Spots	White spots on the buccal mucosa.	Measles
Kussmaul Respirations	Extreme centrally activated hyperventilation (respiratory alkalosis)	Diabetic Ketoacidosis
Kussmaul's Sign	Upon inspiration, finding of an increase in central venous pressure (CVP), rather than a decreased CVP as expected.	Pericardial Effusion is restricting flow to the right ventricle.
Lentigines	Small brown freckle-like lesions on neck and trunk, not increased by sun exposure.	Pulmonic Stenosis, Hypertrophic Cardiomyopathy
Leukorrhea	Clear or white vaginal discharge with faint musty odour.	Pregnancy, other circumstances too
Lid Lag	Evidence of white sclerae between the iris and the upper eyelid, which is normally not present unless the patient actively stares.	Grave's Disease
Macroglossia	Having an enlarged tongue.	Acromegaly, amyloidosis
Malar {Butterfly) Rash	Characteristic rash on cheeks, made worse by UV-light exposure.	Systemic Lupus I Erythematosus (SLE)
Marcus Gunn·Pupil	Pupil dilates rather than constricts when light swings toward it.	Retinopathy: Indicates either severe macular or optic nerve disease in the affected eye.
Miosis	Constricted pupils.	Horner's Syndrome, Opiate Overdose
Moon Facies	Fatty deposits over cheek, thin skin.	Cushing's Syndrome
Murphy's Sign	RUQ pain aggravated by inspiration.	Acute Cholecystitis

Finding	Description, Comments	Associated Disease(s)
Neovascularization	FUNDUSCOPIC: Formation of excess vessels, occurring in response to retinal hypoxia.	Diabetic Retinopathy: Proliferative Retinopathy
Oppenheim's Sign	Scratch inner side of leg ------> extension of toes.	Cerebral Irritation
Osier's Nodes	Tender erythematous nodules on the distal finger-pads.	Infective Endocarditis
Palmomental Reflex	Rub the thenar eminence ------> elicit reflexive contraction of the muscles of the chin.	Frontal Lobe Lesion: A primitive reflex.
Pectus Excavatum (Funnel-Chest)	Sternum curved inward.	Rickets, Marfan Syndrome
Pectus Carinatum (Pigeon Chest)	Increased anteroposterior length of chest. Ribs bowed outward.	Rickets, Marfan Syndrome
Petechiae	Capillary haemorrhages.	Endocarditis: Conjunctival petechiae are seen.
Pingueculae	Small, yellowish elevations of the conjunctivae. It is caused by hyaline degeneration of conjunctival tissue.	Gaucher's Disease: Will see brownish discoloration of Pingueculae.
Psuedomembrane	Whitish, dirty-brown membrane over the tonsils.	Diphtheria
Ptosis	Droopy eyelids. Failure of levator palpebrae muscle to hold up eyelids (innervated by CN III).	Horner's Syndrome, Myasthenia Gravis, Encephalitis
Pulsus Bisferiens (Bifid Pulse)	Two distinct impulses with each heartbeat.	Aortic Insufficiency, Hypertrophic Cardiomyopathy
Pulsus Paradoxus	Upon inspiration, weakening of the arterial pulse by more than expected. Normal decrease in systolic pressure should be 10 mm Hg or less.	Constrictive Pericarditis, Pericardial Effusion, or some other constrictive cardiac condition.

Finding	Description, Comments	Associated Disease(s)
Pulsus Alterans	One pulse feels large, the next pulse feels small.	Congestive Heart Failure (CHF), poor myocardial contractility. Carries a poor prognosis.
Quincke's Pulse	Visible capillary pulsations in the nail-bed.	Aortic Insufficiency
Rhonchus	On auscultation, snoring sound heard over lungs.	Asthma
Romberg Test	Patient can't maintain balance with legs tight together, with eyes closed.	Cerebellar Disease
Roth's Spots	FUNDUSCOPIC: Retinal haemorrhages with pale or white centres.	Infective Endocarditis, Collagen Diseases, Dysproteinemias, Leukemia, Pernicious Anemia
Sausage-shaped fingers	Swelling of the tendon sheath.	Psoriatic Arthritis, Reiter's Syndrome
Simian Crease	Single large horizontal crease on palms.	Down's Syndrome
Strawberry Tongue	Erythematous tongue.	Scarlet Fever
Striae	Red and blue abdominal stretch marks, due to central fat deposits plus thinning skin	Cushing's Syndrome
Subcutaneous Nodules	Granulomatous nodules found over elbows, skull, pr spine. Often associated with cardiac involvement. One of the Major Jones Criteria.	Rheumatic Fever
Succussion Splash	Sounds of gastric activity, normally heard after a large meal.	Pyloric Obstruction: Succussion splash heard after 24 hours of fasting is indicative of pyloric obstruction.
Suck Reflex	Gently tap or rub the upper lift------> elicit a reflexive sucking or puckering response.	Frontal Lobe Lesion: A primitive reflex.

Finding	Description, Comments	Associated Disease(s)
Swan Neck Deformity	Hyperextended PIP joints, plus flexed DIP joints, resulting from subluxation of joints.	Rheumatoid Arthritis
Tinel's Sign	Tingling shots of pain over median nerve upon percussion of the wrist.	Carpel Tunnel Syndrome
Titubatlon	Body tremor when standing or walking.	Cerebellar Disease
Tophi	Nodules of urate deposits can be found anywhere, but usually near joints.	Gout
Trousseau's Sign	Trousseau's Sign. Inflate a blood-pressure cuff to systolic pressure and maintain for 1-2 minutes. Look for induction of carpal spasm.	Tetany
Ulnar Deviation	Deviation of fingers or enter wrist toward ulnar (medial) side.	Rheumatoid Arthritis
Waxy Exudates	FUNDUSCOPIC: Hard lipid-exudates on retina.	Diabetic Retinopathy: Background Retinopathy
Background Retinopathy	On expiration, squeaking high-pitched sound, often audible to unaided ear.	Asthma, Emphysema, COPD
Xanthelasma	Yellow, flat lipid containing lesions around the eyes.	Hyperlipidemia

ILLUSTRATIONS

1.   **PECTUS EXAVATUM**

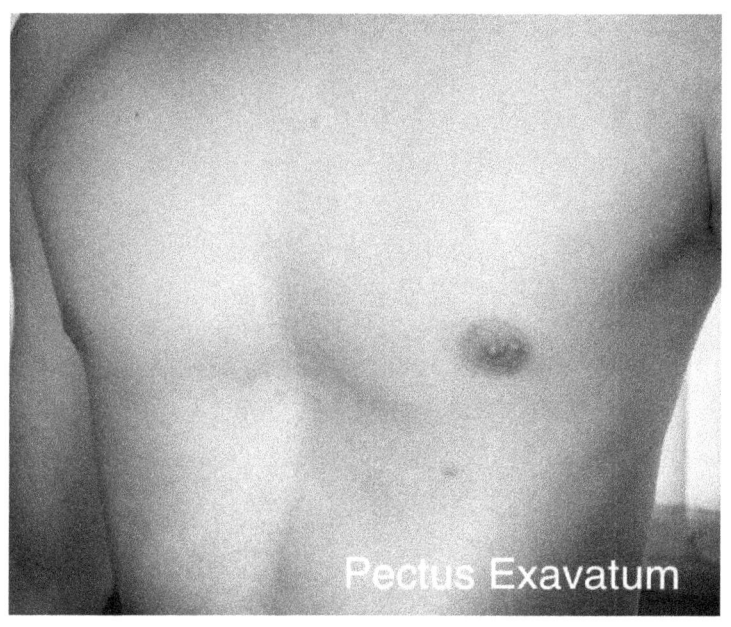

2. MACROGLOSSIA

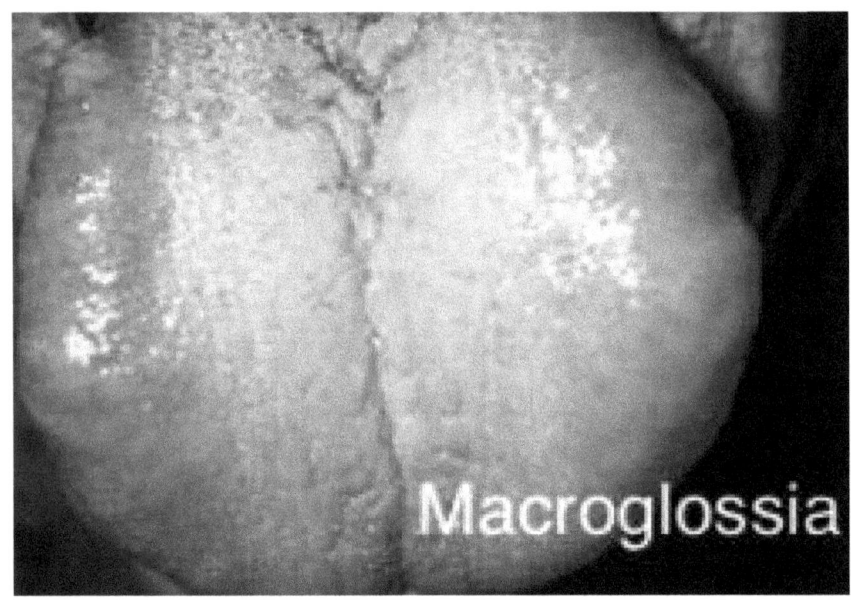

3. CHADDOCK'S SIGN

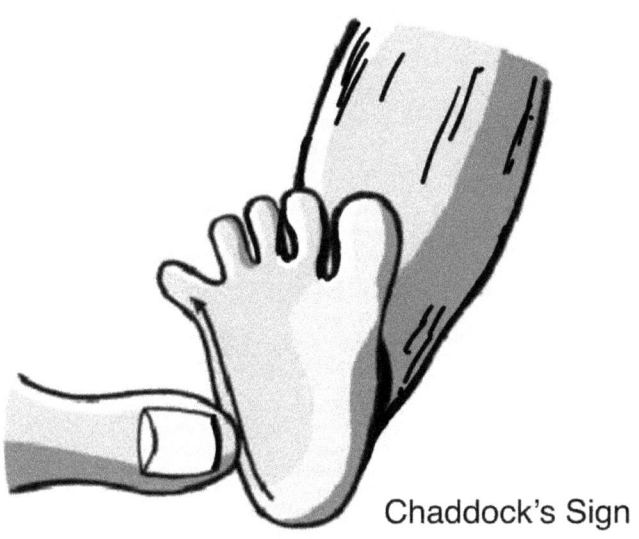

Chaddock's Sign

4. ARCUS SENILIS

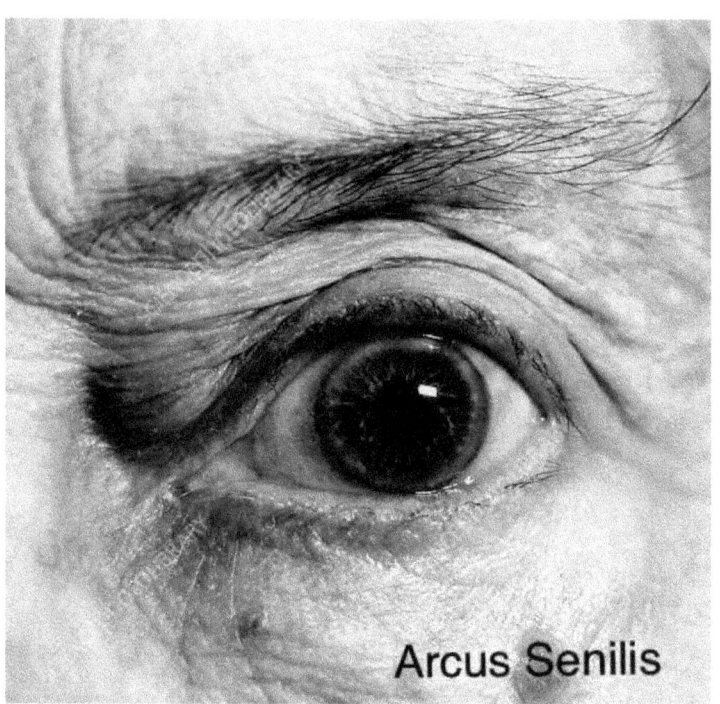

5. CLUBBING

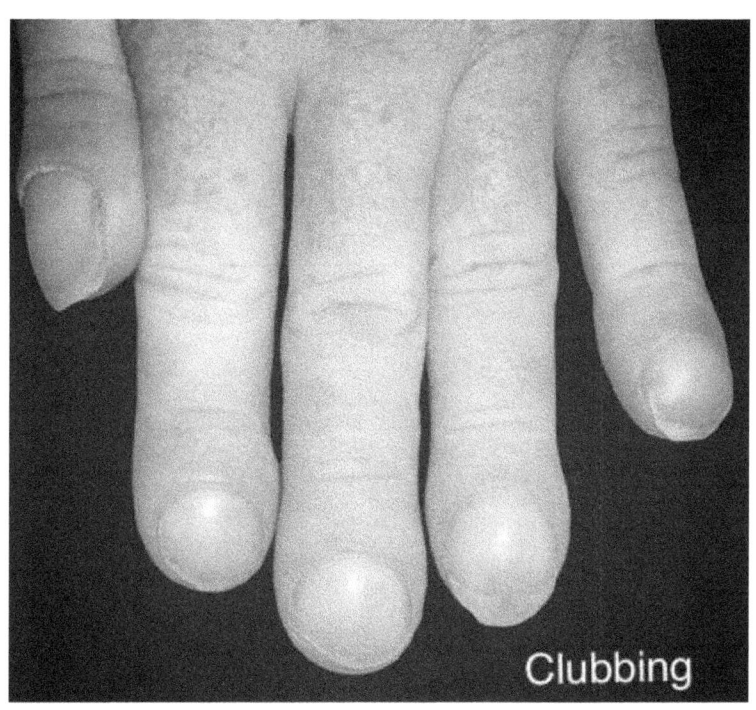

6. **Trousseau Sign**

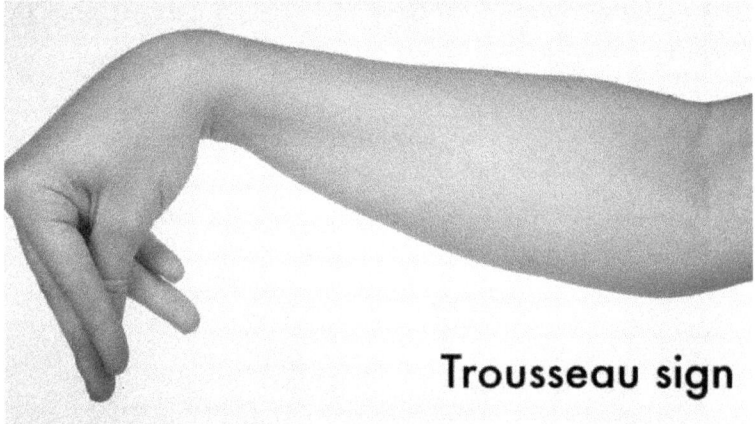

7. EXOPTHALMOS

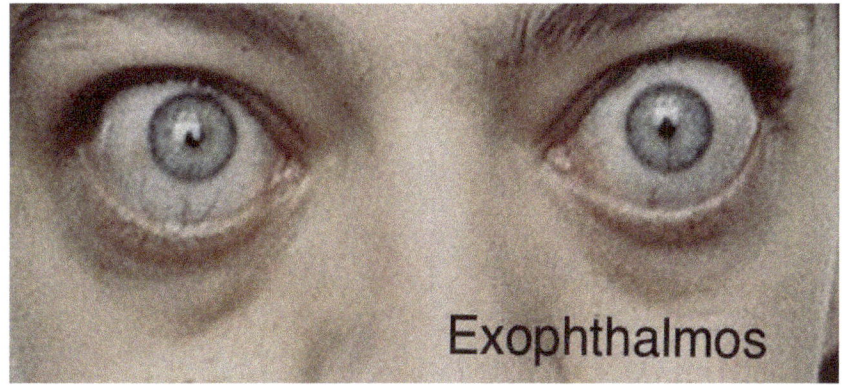

8. ANGIOID STREAKS

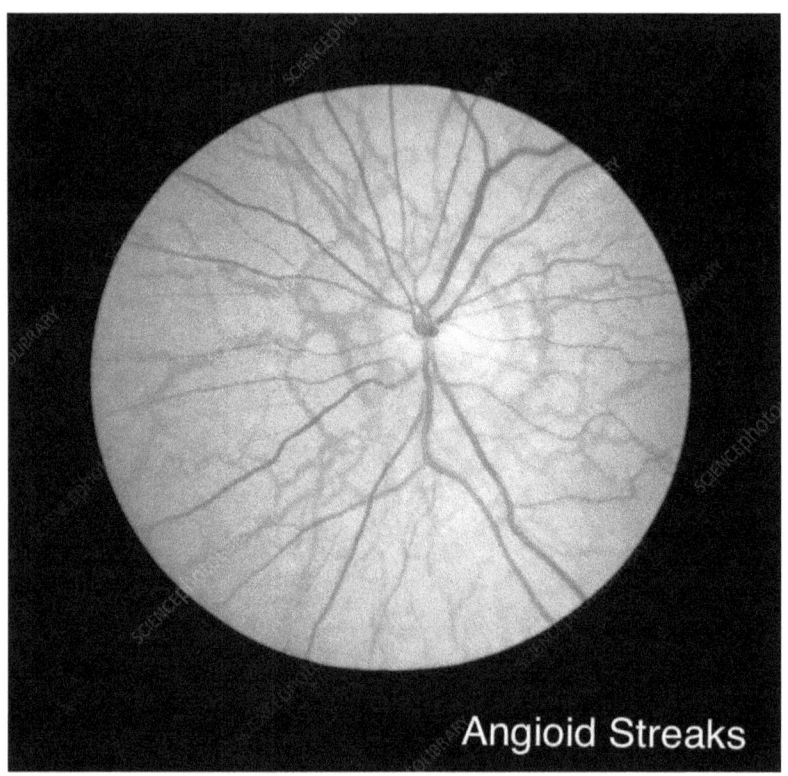

9. CULLEN'S SIGN

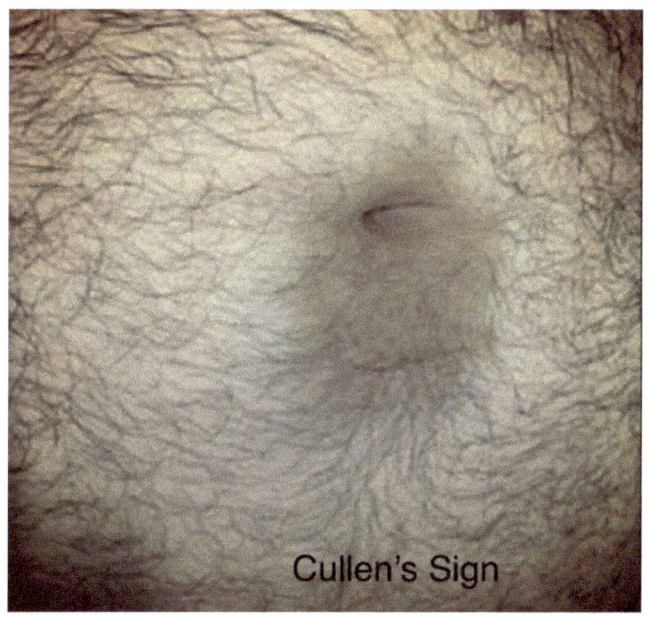

10. COTTONWOOL ESXUDATES

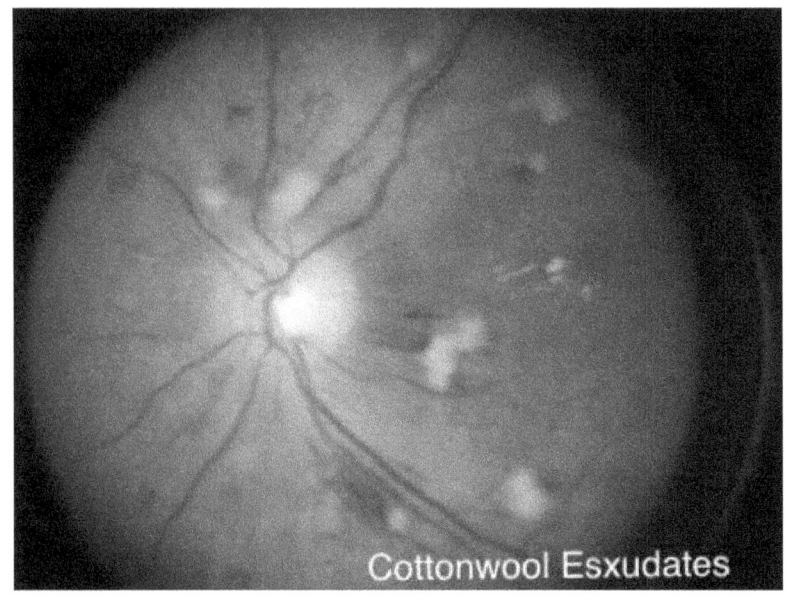

11. Hebberden's Nodules

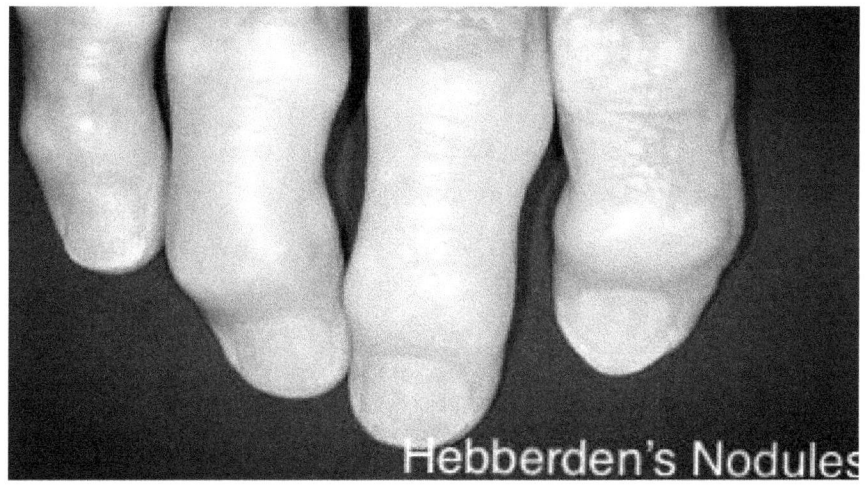

12. Café au Lait spots

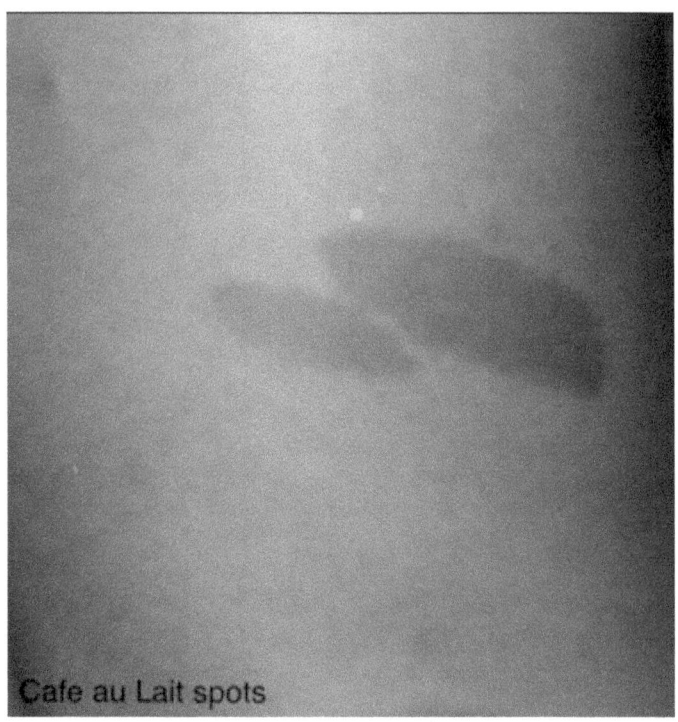

13. GREY TURNER'S SIGN

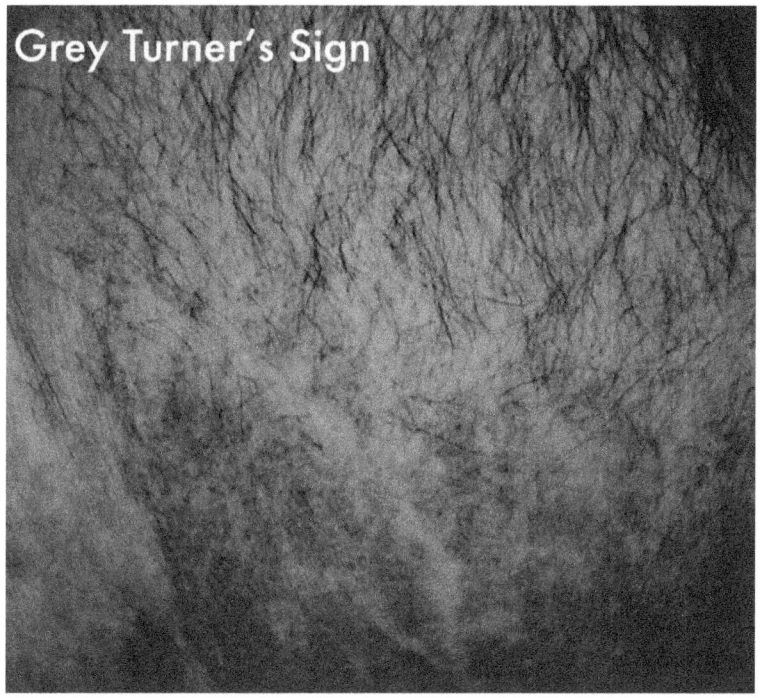

14. Chvostek's sign

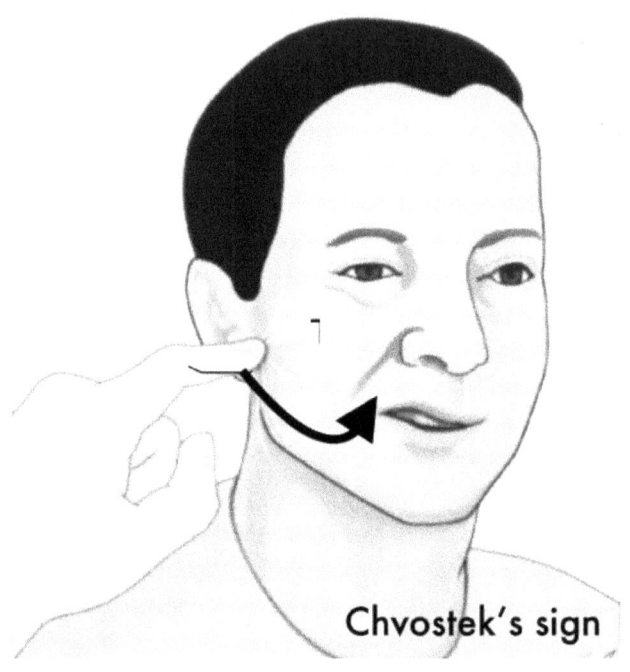

15. SIMIAN CREASE

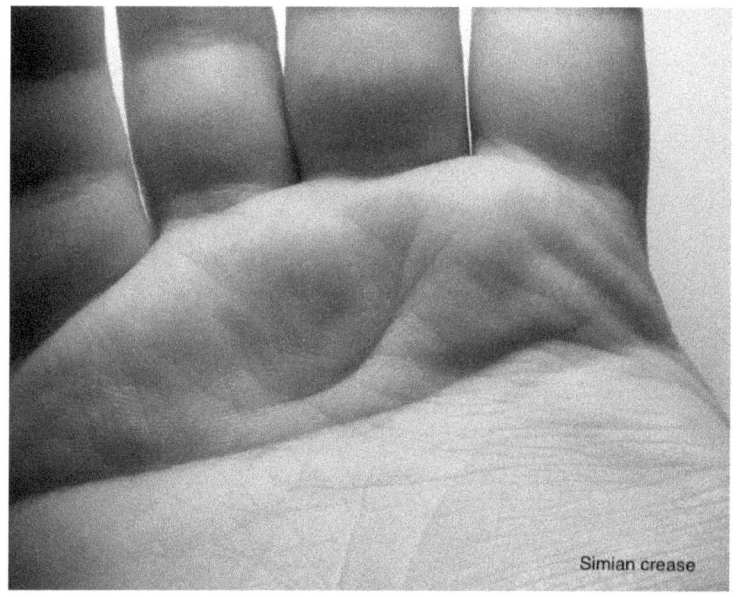

16.　Doll's Eye Movement

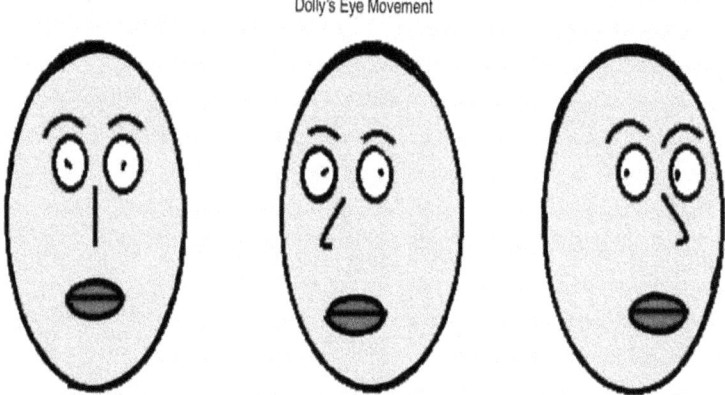
Dolly's Eye Movement

17. KESTENBAUM'S SIGN

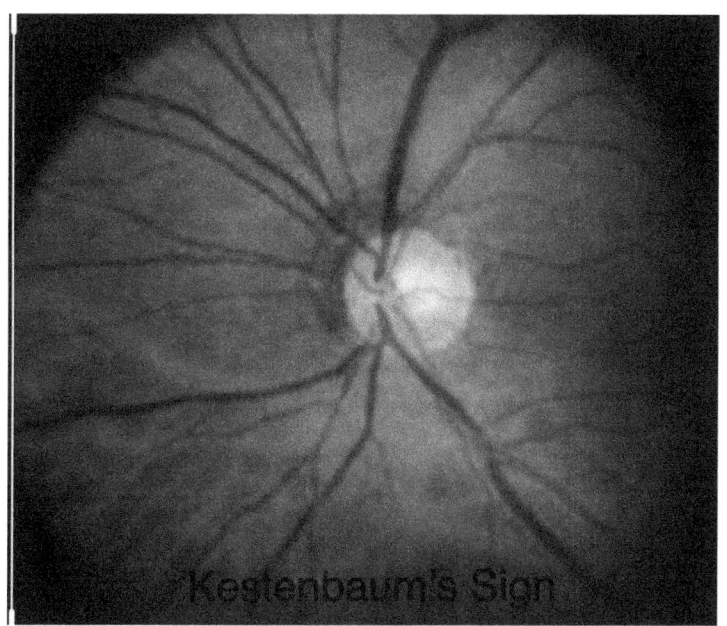

18. SWAN NECK DEFORMITY

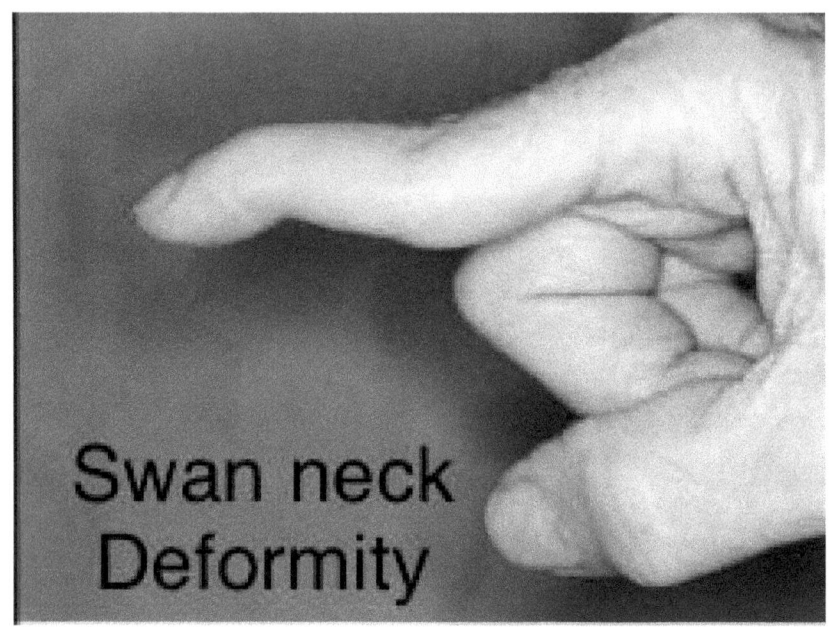

19. PINGUCULAE

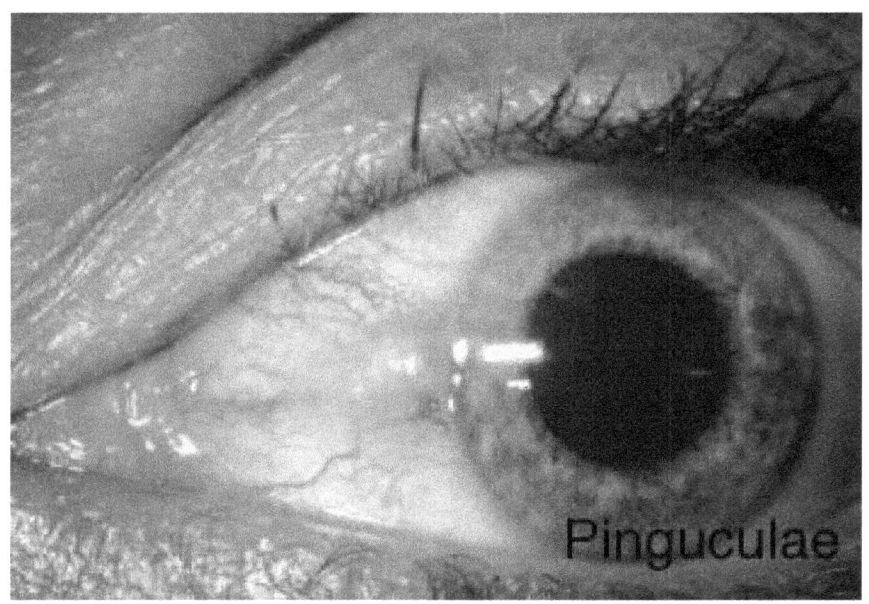

20. DIABETIC RETINOPATHY

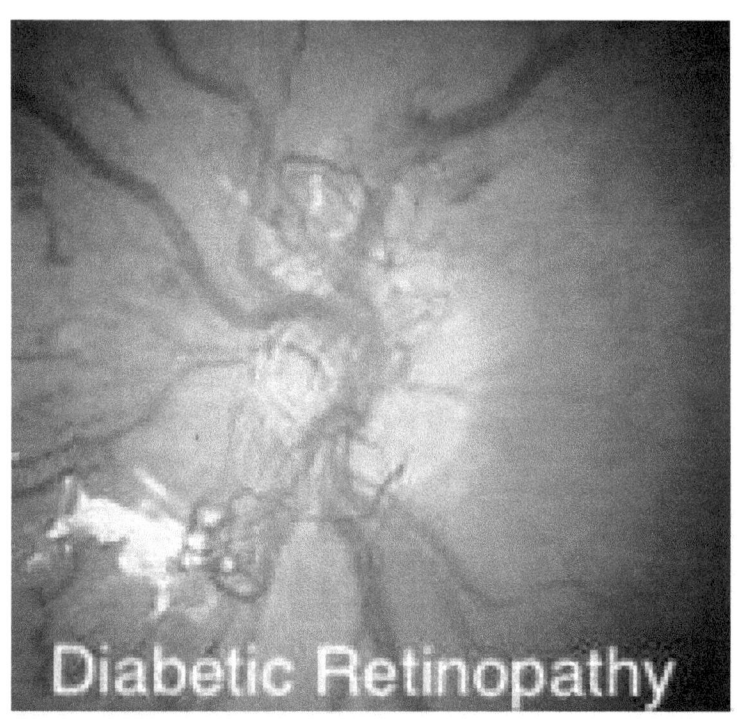

21. BABINSKI SIGN

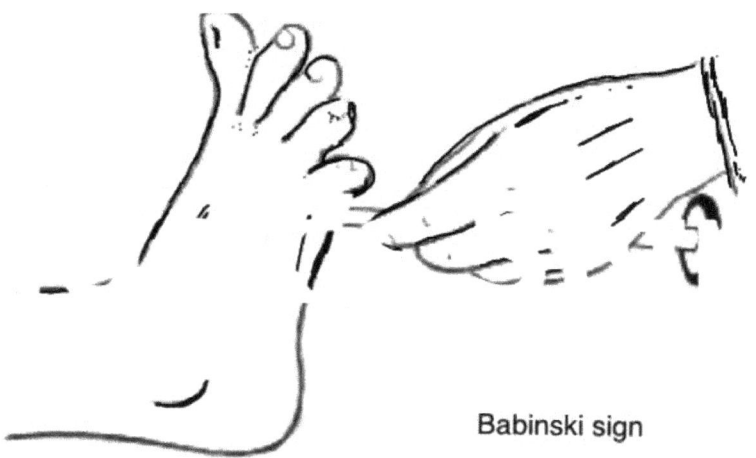

Babinski sign

22. KOPLICK SPOTS

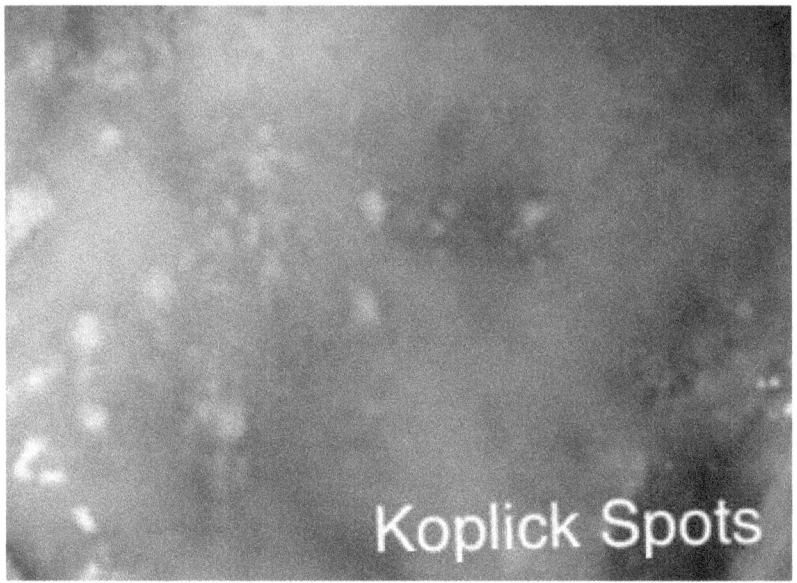

23. BATTLE'S SIGN

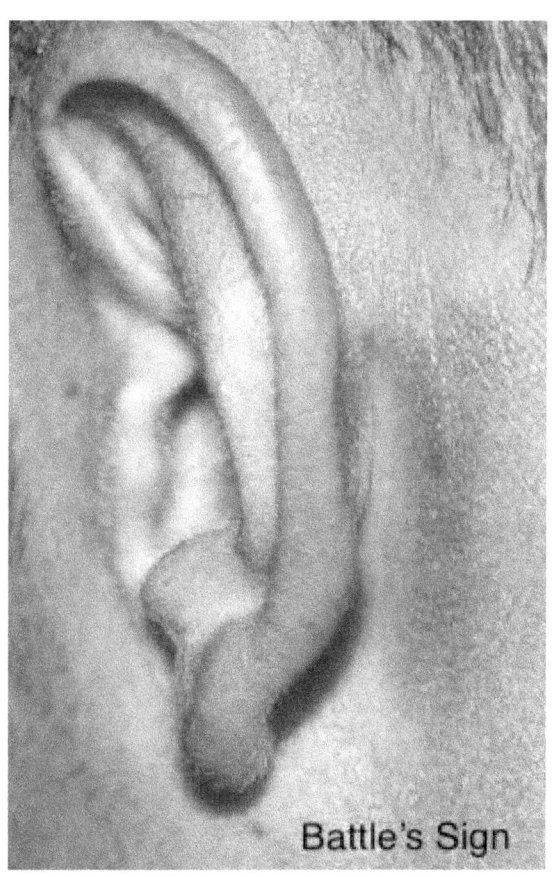

24.   ARGYL ROBERTSON PUPILS

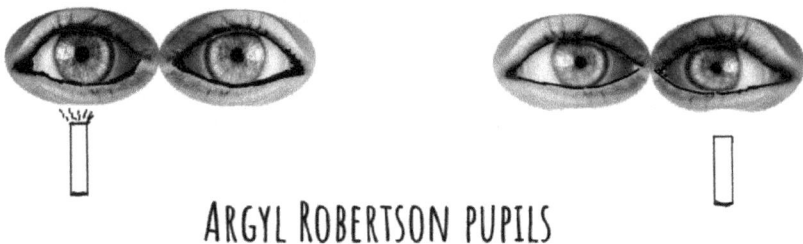

www.ingramcontent.com/pod-product-compliance
Lightning Source LLC
Chambersburg PA
CBHW040521220526
45473CB00013B/2941